SpringerBriefs in Applied Sciences and Technology

PoliMI SpringerBriefs

Series Editors

Barbara Pernici, DEIB, Politecnico di Milano, Milano, Italy

Stefano Della Torre, DABC, Politecnico di Milano, Milano, Italy

Bianca M. Colosimo, DMEC, Politecnico di Milano, Milano, Italy

Tiziano Faravelli, DCHEM, Politecnico di Milano, Milano, Italy

Roberto Paolucci, DICA, Politecnico di Milano, Milano, Italy

Silvia Piardi, Design, Politecnico di Milano, Milano, Italy

Gabriele Pasqui, DASTU, Politecnico di Milano, Milano, Italy

Springer, in cooperation with Politecnico di Milano, publishes the PoliMI Springer-Briefs, concise summaries of cutting-edge research and practical applications across a wide spectrum of fields. Featuring compact volumes of 50 to 125 (150 as a maximum) pages, the series covers a range of contents from professional to academic in the following research areas carried out at Politecnico:

- Aerospace Engineering
- Bioengineering
- Electrical Engineering
- Energy and Nuclear Science and Technology
- Environmental and Infrastructure Engineering
- Industrial Chemistry and Chemical Engineering
- Information Technology
- Management, Economics and Industrial Engineering
- Materials Engineering
- Mathematical Models and Methods in Engineering
- Mechanical Engineering
- Structural Seismic and Geotechnical Engineering
- Built Environment and Construction Engineering
- Physics
- Design and Technologies
- Urban Planning, Design, and Policy

Cinzia Cappiello

Editor

Special Topics in Information Technology

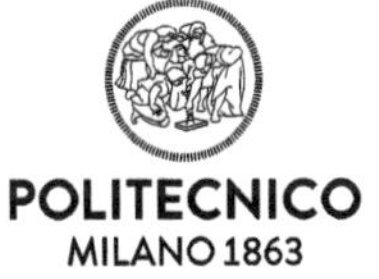

POLITECNICO
MILANO 1863

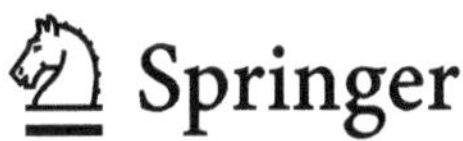
Springer

Editor
Cinzia Cappiello
Dipartimento di Elettronica, Informazione e
Bioingegneria
Politecnico di Milano
Milan, Italy

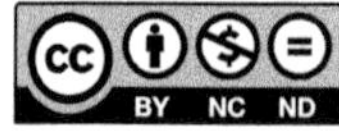

ISSN 2191-530X ISSN 2191-5318 (electronic)
SpringerBriefs in Applied Sciences and Technology
ISSN 2282-2577 ISSN 2282-2585 (electronic)
PoliMI SpringerBriefs
ISBN 978-3-032-12358-9 ISBN 978-3-032-12359-6 (eBook)
https://doi.org/10.1007/978-3-032-12359-6

This work was supported by Politecnico di Milano.

This Springer imprint is published by the registered company Springer Nature Switzerland AG
The registered company address is: Gewerbestrasse 11, 6330 Cham, Switzerland

If disposing of this product, please recycle the paper.

Preface

It is with great pleasure that I present this volume, *Special Topics in Information Technology*, a collection of 12 distinguished contributions authored by Ph.D. students who have completed their doctoral studies in Information Technology at the Dipartimento di Elettronica, Informazione e Bioingegneria of the Politecnico di Milano during the academic year 2024/2025. Carefully selected by the Faculty Board of the Ph.D. Program in Information Technology, they represent approximately the top ten percent of the candidates and stand as a testament to the excellence, creativity, and innovation that define the research conducted within our department.

The Ph.D. program in Information Technology at the Politecnico di Milano has been active for more than 40 years. Its mission is to promote research excellence by encouraging the development of innovative methodologies and cutting-edge technologies, while preparing new generations of researchers and professionals who will advance academic knowledge and drive innovation across industry and society. The Ph.D. program is built on four main areas of study: computer science and engineering, electronics, systems and control, and telecommunications. This structure enables the program to cover an extensive range of research domains within the IT field. The contributions included in this volume provide an inspiring overview of the most significant research achievements in all four of these areas.

While grounded in rigorous scientific methods, the chapters are written in a manner that makes their content accessible to a broad audience, allowing both non-specialists and readers with a more technical background to appreciate the groundbreaking advancements achieved by our Ph.D. students. Each contribution reflects the diversity and depth of the four areas that define our Ph.D. program, showcasing the outstanding quality of the research conducted at our institution and the pivotal role of Information Technology in shaping modern society.

To conclude, I would like to express my gratitude to the contributing authors for their timely and enthusiastic participation in the creation of this volume. It is my hope that it will serve as both a record of their achievements and an inspiration for future generations of researchers.

Milan, Italy   Cinzia Cappiello
October 2025

Contents

Computer Science and Engineering

Machine Learning in Oncogenomics: A Key to Dissecting Cancer Inner Heterogeneity

Silvia Cascianelli

Abstract Computational oncogenomics has a pivotal role to solve biological and clinical issues and support translational medicine in cancer research through computer science and bioinformatics methods. Leveraging advanced computational methods for comprehensive omics analysis is increasingly essential to deepen the understanding of tumor molecular complexity. The research activity outlined in this chapter emphasised the synergistic use of Data Science techniques and omics data processing to tackle clinical challenges of cancer diseases and face their inherent intricacy and heterogeneity. These often pose an insurmountable barrier to traditional research approaches; therefore, we designed and developed computational workflows that follow every step of a typical Data Science process while being enhanced and tailored for omics data, considering all their peculiarities and issues. Overall, this research delivered innovative computational frameworks contributing to unravelling cancer complexity, advancing personalized oncology, and paving the way for precision medicine through comprehensive, clinically driven omics analysis.

1 Motivations and Topics of the Research

In the landscape of cancer research, the combination of high-throughput Next-Generation Sequencing (NGS) technologies with advanced computational methods has ushered in a new era marked by unprecedented research opportunities, challenges and outstanding achievements for computational oncogenomics. Omics data and metadata (i.e., all the clinical/biological annotations) of cancer patients, whose availability is growing dramatically, demand thorough investigations to find answers to unsolved biomedical questions, understand cancer molecular complexity and improve care. Particularly, providing reliable predictions to address relevant patient stratification issues in cancer research is pivotal for medical progress. A fusion of skills and knowledge spanning Computer Science, Data Science, Machine Learning,

S. Cascianelli (✉)
Politecnico di Milano, Department of Electronics, Information and Bioengineering, Milano, Italy
e-mail: silvia.cascianelli@polimi.it

C. Cappiello (ed.), *Special Topics in Information Technology*,
PoliMI SpringerBriefs, https://doi.org/10.1007/978-3-032-12359-6_1

Bioinformatics, and Oncogenomics is therefore essential to obtain robust results and solutions for computational oncogenomics problems. Yet, to date, the application of Data Science (DS) techniques and, particularly, Machine Learning (ML) models in Oncogenomics has mostly been constrained by two main approaches. A tendency to treat omics data merely as complex input for ML algorithms, without considering the peculiar characteristics of the data and tasks involved. A tendency to apply ML methods without the needed expertise or the establishment of rigorous pipelines.

In this research, fully-legit DS workflows, including steps of rigorous omics data processing, ML model development and performance assessment, were merged with clinical validation and interpretability efforts to strengthen computational findings with clear biological evidence. Collaborations with experts in Medicine and Biology steered the research activity towards hot topics in Oncogenomics, aligning with real translational needs and noteworthy applications to breast and colorectal cancer, where the efficacy of the proposed methods was confirmed. Great attention was devoted to omics data exploration and integration, as well as to the feature engineering and selection phase. Advanced computing methods were used to analyze different cancer omics data and dig into the expression patterns, alterations and mutations driving cancer differentiation and response to treatment. Predictive modelling and result evaluation were tailored to face the issues of oncogenomics research scenarios and provide interpretation and validation from both computational and clinical-biological perspectives, as further discussed in this chapter.

The research was first directed to the enhancement of an R/Bioconductor package designed for efficient investigation and integration of omics data [1]. Then, we achieved remarkable methodological advances in cancer patient stratifications, as proved by successful applications to breast (BRCA) and colorectal (CRC) cancer. These include defining a new feature selection method to tackle unbalanced classification scenarios [2]; investigating multi-omics, deep and semi-supervised solutions in light of the increasing omics data availability [3]; transitioning towards multi-label transcriptional classification of patients to better reflect the underlying molecular heterogeneity of each patient [4, 5]. Lastly, innovative mutation-based feature engineering and supervised multi-omics frameworks were combined with variant prioritisation approaches and search for actionable genes to find new potential therapeutic targets for cancer patient groups of critical medical handling [6, 7].

Overall, this research activity aimed to design and implement reproducible DS investigations to study cancer inner heterogeneity, provide clinically relevant insights and stratifications for single patients affected by different types of cancer and identify genes, variants and models with therapeutic and prognostic value. A systematic procedural approach was employed to address each research question related to different cancer stratification scenarios. All the stages of a DS life cycle were performed (*Problem Definition, Data Collection, Data Cleaning, Data Exploration, Predictive Modelling, Result delivery*), organising each research in the following key phases:

- Retrieval and processing of omics datasets and their metadata, mainly from public sources.

- Deep study of state-of-the-art methods and clinical tests, improvement or ex-novo ML implementation.
- Design and development of clinically relevant Omics DS solutions using unsupervised, supervised or semi-supervised ML approaches.
- Comparative performance evaluation of all the considered approaches, refinements to ensure robustness and interpretability and analysis of the omics features playing the main roles.
- Validation of models and results by assessing biological and clinical value against the available metadata.

Consequently, significant methodological and application contributions were provided, including the relevant examples presented in the following sections.

2   Enhancing Cancer Subtyping Methods

Traditionally, cancer subtyping methods have been focused mainly on transcriptomics and, particularly, on the analysis of limited sets of gene expression profiles used to classify patients into distinct molecular subtypes of the affecting primary tumor. Also, the majority of the state-of-the-art subtyping approaches use dataset-level similarity-based methods [8–15], leveraging various correlation or distance metrics to classify an entire patient cohort and non-fully standardized procedures and dataset-dependent normalization, which imply limitations in terms of reproducibility and usage for individual samples. ML-based subtyping approaches solve these main limitations [16], offering fully-reproducible single-sample classification technique for patient stratification.

However, a critical challenge to address in cancer subtyping tasks is the elevated sensitivity of ML models to high feature cardinality and variability. Several existing feature selection approaches were already adopted for expression-based cancer subtyping (e.g., [16–18]), and many approaches were proposed from the early stage of genomic advent to address the need for predictive gene signatures [19]. Nonetheless, the increasing availability of NGS data counting up to a hundred thousand genes per sample, led to the pressing demand for new efficient and effective selection strategies. NGS omics data, with their huge feature space sizes and growing sample volumes, exhibit big data characteristics, whilst they still maintain a disproportion between sample availability (especially samples with multi-omics profiles) and feature dimensions. Furthermore, subtyping problems are also often hindered by the high imbalance in sample distribution among the classes of interest, which reflects the real occurrence of cases. Thus, achieving proper cancer patient stratification represents a critical challenge. Feature selection strategies able to extract useful predictive features by removing irrelevant, redundant, and noisy ones are crucial to achieving valuable, robust results on a desired NGS-based subtyping task. Furthermore, accounting for the strongly unbalanced class distribution plays a key role in improving the reliability even for smaller classes.

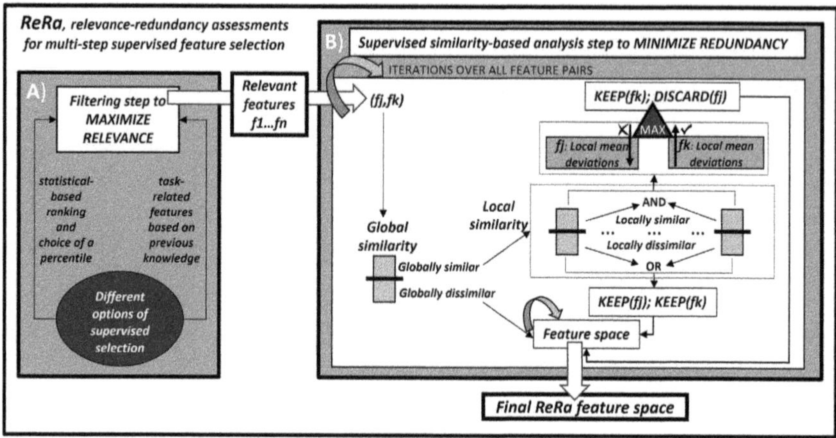

Fig. 1 Flowchart with the two steps of the supervised maximum relevance minimum redundancy feature selection approach, named ReRa. Adapted from [2]

Accordingly, we designed and developed an innovative feature selection approach named ReRa, which uses two sequential steps of RElevance and Redundancy Assessments to preserve significantly differentiated features for predictive performance improvement while considering the class imbalance of the desired classification tasks. Its main steps are summarized in Fig. 1. Its feature relevance estimation step enables exploring and comparing several options (e.g., statistical and knowledge-based filtering) in the awareness that some are more suitable than others for a given task. However, the main strength of this approach is unveiling potential class-specific divergences between feature pairs that are overlooked from a global perspective (e.g. by a Maximum Relevance Minimum Redundancy algorithm—MRmr [20]) but may contribute to improving class distinction. In fact, in the redundancy elimination step, ReRa leverages not only global but also class-specific similarity assessments based on supervised training labels. This guarantees to distinguish true redundant features, which are minimized, from features globally similar across all samples, but well-differentiated 'locally', i.e., within one or more specific classes. Furthermore, its iterative redundancy minimization procedure reevaluates and updates the selected features at each iteration without employing a fixed, growing subset and without the need for specifying a feature space size to reach. Preserving class-differentiated features, ReRa not only improves the performance of ML models in highly unbalanced classification tasks but also provides insights into distinctive omics features and molecular traits of each class, a key aspect for translational applications like cancer subtyping.

Remarkably, ReRa demonstrated superior performance compared to conventional methods such as filters, embedded regularizations or MRmr [20] in two different NGS-based BRCA subtyping scenarios, one at the gene and isoform transcriptomics level. This comparative analysis demonstrated the power of ReRa without compromising the generalizability of the approach to face various feature types and tasks of interest. Indeed, the role of ReRa can be central to investigating class differentiation even in more complex omics spaces like isoforms or even genotypes, as more recently proven in [21], enhancing our understanding of patient subtypes and therapeutic implications.

3 Transitioning Towards Multi-label Cancer Subtyping

Though traditional cancer subtyping is crucial in biomedical research and clinical practice, using single-label classification methods may simplify the molecular portrait of a tumor, overlooking the inner complexity and the co-existence of multiple class traits. Research has recently suggested these subtypes could denote phenotypic states with potential overlap rather than discrete, mutually exclusive states [22]. Accordingly, this research activity emphasized the importance of investigating multi-label subtyping to better dissect cancer inner heterogeneity. Starting from the transcriptional level, the transition to comprehensive multi-label subtyping allowed us to capture a full molecular landscape of individual patients and paved the way for improved predictions for patients in diverse disease contexts.

Multi-label strategies, able to associate each patient with more than one subtype, had barely been addressed so far in relevant translational applications like cancer subtyping. Consequently, supervised multi-label information was missing to learn multi-label classification tasks directly. In our work, alternative strategies were therefore designed and implemented to move towards multi-label classification in cancer subtyping, including:

- A tailored problem adaptation strategy to transform single-label models into multi-label adapted classifiers without the need for multi-label example data for the training phase;
- A two-step workflow to first provide multi-label sample characterization for model training (extending similarity-based methods), and then, find the most promising multi-label classification solution for a given task;
- An integrative approach for comprehensive cancer stratification combining unsupervised clustering, transfer learning, regression models and multi-label predictions, currently under a patent application process.

These strategies represent noteworthy methodological contributions of this research activity and were employed in corresponding DS investigations to: assess for the first time the relevance of multi-label characterization in colorectal cancer subtyping; offer a generalizable workflow for multi-label stratification of a given disease, as already verified on breast and colorectal cancer subtyping; enhance colorectal cancer intrinsic subtyping by addressing current limitations in its classification. From each of these investigations, we provided valuable multi-label predictors demonstrating that the clinical value of predicting both primary and secondary assignments for each patient overcomes that of predicting the primary assignments only. Furthermore, we showed that assessing and interpreting differences and similarities among patients sharing multiple subtype assignments (either partially or totally) is crucial to obtaining more appropriate cancer patient descriptions and better clinical/therapeutic indications.

Specifically, the objective of our first DS investigation on CRC was to assess whether assigning multiple CRIS subtypes (i.e. intrinsic molecular subtypes derived from [10]) to a single sample could yield additional clinically and biologically relevant insights, and reflect underlying tumour cell population heterogeneity. Towards this aim, we developed a tailored algorithm-adaptation strategy to obtain multi-label ML-based subtyping models from simpler single-label classification models. Specifically, training a supervised model of interest for single-label subtyping task version implies to compute for each of the training samples a score with respect to every class before assigning the sample to its own class through a softmax transformation. The softmax transformation at the end of a classification pipeline is meant to strengthen the algorithm in returning a single class (i.e. its 'primary', most prominent class). However, all the class scores computed before the softmax transformation can estimate how much a sample belongs to any class. Thus, in order to possibly assign one or more additional 'secondary' classes to a sample based on its class scores, our strategy required calculating for every classifier class-specific score thresholds through the following approach. First, we extracted the class scores produced by the single-label classifier without using its final softmax layer. Then, the scores for each sample were independently normalized class-by-class to a [0, 1] range, using the min and max score values of each class in the training dataset. This normalization was used to obtain comparable class membership values for each sample. Always considering training samples only, we took the distributions of these normalized membership values grouped by class, and from each distribution, we obtained a class-specific threshold as the class mean value diminished by 2.5 times the class coefficient of variation. By means of these thresholds, we were able to capture samples associated with a class also when it is not the primary class. If an unseen test sample had a normalized class score greater or equal to the corresponding class-specific threshold, the multi-label adapted algorithm would assign the sample to that class. Notice the class-specific thresholds and scaling parameters did not invalidate the purpose of obtaining single-sample classifiers, since they were pre-computed on training data, only during the threshold definition phase, and were then simply applied to independent testing data without further modifications.

Through this algorithm adaptation strategy, multi-label adapted versions of many distinct single-label classifiers were made available to assign unseen CRC samples, not only with their primary classes but possibly with multi-label assignments. The classification performances obtained on a CRC dataset of testing demonstrated the efficacy and reliability of this approach and of the obtained multi-label classifiers. Particularly, after a wide comparative assessment, the best classification solution appeared to be a multi-label adapted linear Support Vector Machine, made available as ML^2CRIS predictor for CRC, as reported in the work published on Genome

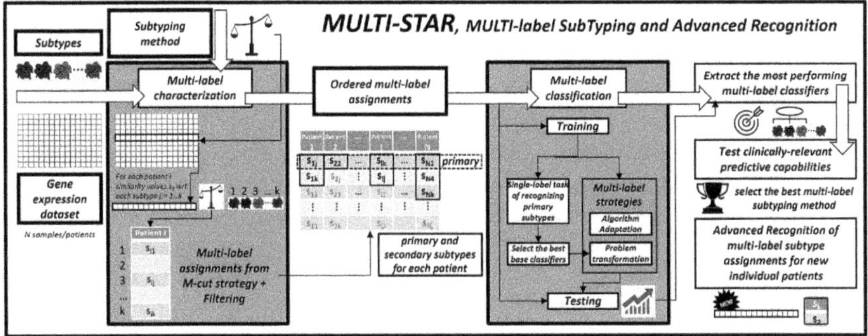

Fig. 2 Schematic description of the MULTI-STAR workflow with its two consecutive steps of multi-label characterization and multi-label classification. Adapted from [5]

Medicine [4]. ML^{2}CRIS demonstrated its capability of capturing inner heterogeneity of any individual CRC patient, as required in clinics. By shedding light on previously overlooked secondary assignments, it unveiled that multi-label patient stratifications are definitely more accurate, prognostically relevant and useful for clinical handling and therapeutic decision processes.

Nonetheless, to address the shortcomings of the existing similarity-based transcriptional subtyping methods and obtain machine learning-based multi-label classifiers without the need for tailored adaptation strategies and processing, we also designed an easy-to-use computational workflow named MULTI-STAR (MULTI-label SubTyping and Advanced Recognition). MULTI-STAR approach, as depicted in Fig. 2, serves a dual purpose for any specific subtyping task at hand:

- Establish a comprehensive supervised reference of *multi-label characterization* for the training samples, by leveraging and extending a similarity-based subtyping method at the state-of-the-art;
- Optimize the most promising *multi-label classification* methods, obtained supervisely using the *multi-label characterizations* results and evaluating alternative multi-label strategies of problem transformation and algorithm adaptation.

MULTI-STAR-based classifiers provide advanced recognition of all the subtypes that influence a patient's molecular and clinical profile, providing a complete multi-label characterization but distinguishing the primary subtype from additional relevant secondary ones. Their effectiveness was demonstrated in multi-label BRCA and CRC subtyping, where they overcame existing approaches in prognostic performance, particularly for survival predictions, while analyzing each sample independently, as required in clinical practice. Given the complexity of the multi-label classification task, especially in cancer subtyping, where dealing with the absence of patients already associated with multiple labels, the evaluation of each model passed through: an exhaustive performance comparison, including existing label-based and example-based metrics and newly defined measures, that we designed to consider both primary or secondary assignments and their ordering; an in-depth comparison of prognostic capabilities based on the obtained multi-label classifications, considering also secondary assignments. These evaluations underlined the impact of the MULTI-STAR workflow and its derived multi-label models in advancing the field of subtyping towards more precise personalized medicine, as discussed in [5]. Furthermore, by eliminating the need for ad-hoc adaptation strategies, the MULTI-STAR approach streamlined the process of multi-label classifier development, easing future application to different subtyping scenarios, involving different omics data or different heterogeneous diseases.

4   Conclusions

Overall, this reasearch activity focused on developing innovative computational workflows integrating Data Science techniques, especially Machine Learning models, with omics data processing, to target the molecular heterogeneity of cancer, also relying on close collaborations with experts in Medicine and Biology. From both computational and application perspectives, the strategies and workflows developed can provide researchers with robust methodological resources, noteworthy investigations and clinically relevant insights into cancer heterogeneity, while also supporting clinicians with approaches for patient stratification and gene role prioritization.

All the findings contributed to answering open questions in cancer research and shaping new trajectories for precision medicine. Particularly, a fundamental assumption was widely confirmed: cancer diseases are not monolithic entities but are better represented by diverse molecular subtypes, traceable at different omics levels and characterized by their peculiar traits. Hence, importantly, DS investigations and ML methods can offer a valuable refined lens to discern this heterogeneity, enabling reliable identification and prediction of all the clinically relevant subtypes for patient stratifications. Therefore, as the field evolves, training and empowering omics data scientists with interdisciplinary expertise will be crucial to tackle competently the increasing research, technological, and computational demands needed to guide translational research and precision medicine towards new horizons.

References

1. S. Pallotta, S. Cascianelli, M. Masseroli, RGMQL: scalable and interoperable computing of heterogeneous omics big data and metadata in r/bioconductor. BMC Bioinform. **23**(1), 1–28 (2022)
2. S. Cascianelli, A. Galzerano, M. Masseroli, Supervised relevance-redundancy assessments for feature selection in omics-based classification scenarios. J. Biomed. Inf. **144**, 1–12 (2023)

3. F. Cristovao, S. Cascianelli, A. Canakoglu et al., Investigating deep learning based breast cancer subtyping using pan-cancer and multi-omic data. IEEE/ACM Trans. Comput. Biol. Bioinform. **19**(1), 121–134 (2020)
4. S. Cascianelli, C. Barbera, A.A. Ulla, E. Grassi, B. Lupo, D. Pasini, A. Bertotti, L. Trusolino, E. Medico, C. Isella et al., Multi-label transcriptional classification of colorectal cancer reflects tumor cell population heterogeneity. Genome Med. **15**(1), 1–37 (2023)
5. S. Cascianelli, I. Milojkovic, M. Masseroli, A novel machine learning-based workflow to capture intra-patient heterogeneity through transcriptional multi-label characterization and clinically relevant classification. J. Biomed. Inf. **166**, 104817 (2025)
6. S. Cascianelli, C. Iudica, M. Masseroli, A data science approach to investigate the mutational landscape of a critical patient subgroup, in *Proceedings of the 19th International Conference on Computational Intelligence Methods for Bioinformatics and Biostatistics, CIBB 2024*, pp. 1–6 (2024)
7. S. Cascianelli, C. Iudica, M. Masseroli, Three-stage data science methodology to explore genetic heterogeneity of diseases, in *Computational Intelligence Methods for Bioinformatics and Biostatistics*, ed. by L. Cerulo, F. Napolitano, F. Bardozzo, L. Cheng, A. Occhipinti, S.M. Pagnotta (Cham), pp. 150–164 (Springer Nature Switzerland, 2025)
8. S. Biade, M. Marinucci, J. Schick, D. Roberts, G. Workman, E. Sage, P. O'Dwyer, V. Livolsi, S. Johnson, Gene expression profiling of human ovarian tumours. British J. Cancer **95**(8), 1092–1100 (2006)
9. J.S. Parker, M. Mullins, M.C. Cheang, S. Leung, D. Voduc, T. Vickery, S. Davies, C. Fauron, X. He, Z. Hu et al., Supervised risk predictor of breast cancer based on intrinsic subtypes. J. Clin. Oncol. **27**(8), 1160 (2009)
10. C. Isella, F. Brundu, S.E. Bellomo, F. Galimi, E. Zanella, R. Porporato, C. Petti, A. Fiori, F. Orzan, R. Senetta et al., Selective analysis of cancer-cell intrinsic transcriptional traits defines novel clinically relevant subtypes of colorectal cancer. Nat. Commun. **8**(1), 15107 (2017)
11. J. Guinney, R. Dienstmann, X. Wang, A. De Reynies, A. Schlicker, C. Soneson, L. Marisa, P. Roepman, G. Nyamundanda, P. Angelino et al., The consensus molecular subtypes of colorectal cancer. Nat. Med. **21**(11), 1350–1356 (2015)
12. A. Schlicker, G. Beran, C.M. Chresta, G. McWalter, A. Pritchard, S. Weston, S. Runswick, S. Davenport, K. Heathcote, D.A. Castro et al., Subtypes of primary colorectal tumors correlate with response to targeted treatment in colorectal cell lines. BMC Med. Genom. **5**(1), 1–15 (2012)
13. M. Ringnér, G. Jönsson, J. Staaf, Prognostic and chemotherapy predictive value of gene-expression phenotypes in primary lung adenocarcinoma. Clin. Cancer Res. **22**(1), 218–229 (2016)
14. X. Dai, T. Li, Z. Bai, Y. Yang, X. Liu, J.-W. Zhan, B. Shi, Breast cancer intrinsic subtype classification, clinical use and future trends. Am. J. Cancer Res. **5**(10), 2929–2943 (2015)
15. J. Holm, L. Eriksson, A. Ploner, M. Eriksson, M. Rantalainen, J. Li, P. Hall, K. Czene, Assessment of breast cancer risk factors reveals subtype heterogeneity. Cancer Res. **77**(13), 3708–3717 (2017)
16. S. Cascianelli, I. Molineris, C. Isella, M. Masseroli, E. Medico, Machine learning for RNA sequencing-based intrinsic subtyping of breast cancer. Sci. Rep. **10**(1), 1–13 (2020)
17. R.K. Singh, M. Sivabalakrishnan, Feature selection of gene expression data for cancer classification: a review. Procedia Comput. Sci. **50**, 52–57 (2015)
18. S. Mongardi, S. Cascianelli, M. Masseroli, Biologically weighted lasso: Enhancing functional interpretability in gene expression data analysis. *Bioinformatics*, p. btae605 (2024)
19. M. Vahmiyan, M. Kheirabadi, E. Akbari, Feature selection methods in microarray gene expression data: a systematic mapping study. Neural Comput. Appl. **34**(22), 19675–19702 (2022)
20. C. Ding, H. Peng, Minimum redundancy feature selection from microarray gene expression data. J. Bioinform. Comput. Biol. **3**(2), 185–205 (2005)
21. S. Tomè, S. Cascianelli, E. Salvi, and M. Masseroli, Benchmark study on supervised relevance-redundancy assessment for feature selection in genomic data, in *Proceedings of the 19th*

International Conference on Computational Intelligence Methods for Bioinformatics and Biostatistics, CIBB 2024, pp. 1–6 (2024)
22. L. Marisa, Y. Blum, J. Taieb, M. Ayadi, C. Pilati, K. Le Malicot, C. Lepage, R. Salazar, D. Aust, A. Duval et al., Intratumor CMS heterogeneity impacts patient prognosis in localized colon cancer. Clin. Cancer Res. **27**(17), 4768–4780 (2021)

Engaging People with Intellectual Disabilities in IoT Prototyping: Design Guidelines for Accessible Making Toolkits

Diego Morra

Abstract Despite the growing potential of Internet of Things (IoT) technologies to support autonomy and inclusion, individuals with intellectual disabilities (ID) remain largely excluded from the processes of ideating and personalizing these systems. Drawing on results of participatory design studies conducted with three different toolkits, this paper presents findings from a user-centered research involving people with ID in IoT ideation and making. The results are synthesized into a set of design guidelines for accessible toolkit development, with a focus on fostering understanding, agency, and engagement. Furthermore, results emphasize the value of hybrid tangible-digital interactions in addressing physical and cognitive challenges. This paper contributes to the growing body of research on accessible computing by providing empirical evidence and actionable guidelines to democratize access to complex technical domains.

1 Introduction

The Internet of Things (IoT) holds promise for improving the quality of life by enabling personalized smart environments. Recent advancements in co-design and making toolkits have heightened interest among HCI researchers in involving vulnerable communities in technology design, empowering them to become active participants [4]. Based on the documented benefits that young user inclusion in technology making can have on digital well-being [9], including marginalized groups in these processes could lead to similarly significant benefits, unlocking new opportunities for innovation. However, while including young people in technology design is already complex, engaging individuals with ID presents substantial challenges. People with ID may present difficulties with decision-making, complex reasoning, and fine motor coordination. These challenges make conventional technology design and programming activities challenging.

D. Morra (✉)
DEIB Politecnico di Milano, Milan, Italy
e-mail: diego.morra@polimi.it

© The Author(s) 2026

C. Cappiello (ed.), *Special Topics in Information Technology*,
PoliMI SpringerBriefs, https://doi.org/10.1007/978-3-032-12359-6_2

This paper presents the design, development, and validation of a novel toolkit intended to engage individuals with ID in the co-design and prototyping of IoT devices. The proposed toolkit is the result of an iterative research process and builds upon insights derived from prior user studies involving two earlier toolkits. These preliminary studies explored solutions to support participation, comprehension, and agency in IoT design for individuals with ID. The empirical findings from these investigations informed the design rationale of the current toolkit, which integrates phygital (physical and digital) interfaces, tangible components, and simplified interactions to accommodate both cognitive and motor challenges. Through results from user-centered design and a comprehensive user study, this paper investigates the role of accessible making toolkits in democratizing access to IoT making and prototyping for people with ID. Key design guidelines and broader implications for Human-Computer Interaction (HCI) and inclusive technology design are discussed, highlighting how tangible, collaborative approaches can foster empowerment and help reduce the digital divide for people with ID.

2 Background and Related Work

Prior work in assistive technology and educational toolkits has focused on diverse disabilities by adapting physical construction kits or interfaces. However, there are currently limited applications that address the needs of the neurodiverse population [1]. Bridging the gap in making smart device prototyping more accessible and engaging for individuals with ID remains a crucial objective [15]. Including marginalized groups in technology design activities can yield significant benefits, providing a conducive environment, enabling them to exert control and make choices based on their experiences and preferences [14]. Such engagement fosters a sense of ownership and acknowledgment and enhances creativity, teamwork, and social skills [14]. Yet, designing accessible tools for ID population requires careful consideration, starting from supporting the specific needs of this user group while ensuring meaningful participation.

Diverse studies have explored using technology to support individuals with ID, aiming to enhance their cognitive, behavioral, social, and sensory-motor skills [11]. One innovative approach is the development of *phygital* interfaces [6], which combine digital and physical experiences. This approach acknowledges the importance of embodiment in developing cognitive skills such as mental imagery, memory, reasoning, and problem-solving. By integrating physical and digital components, phygital interfaces facilitate physical interaction, physical-to-digital correlations, and multi-sensory engagement, which enhances sensory and educational experiences by combining computational elements with tangible materials [5].

Similarly, adopting Tangible User Interfaces (TUIs) has shown positive outcomes in engagement, collaboration, and initiative [7]. Adopting TUI-based tools inside technology-making activities dedicated to individuals with ID could improve inclusion and participation, fostering independent exploratory and collaborative learning.

In recent years, simplified electronics toolkits have gained momentum, especially in contemporary educational practices, promoting an understanding of electronics and computational thinking across diverse learner populations [12]. These toolkits are crafted to be intuitive, affordable, and accessible, making them well-suited for use in educational environments. They provide hands-on, practical experiences that simplify complex electronic concepts, enhancing engagement and inclusivity in learning and making. However, only a few works from the literature have specifically targeted the creation of toolkits tailored for individuals with ID [3, 15].

2.1 Prior Work with Accessible Toolkits

The research presented in this paper builds on insights from two prior studies investigating the use of tangible, phygital toolkits designed to support individuals with ID in engaging with IoT concepts and design practices.

The first study explored a card-based toolkit named COBO [2], which aimed to investigate how people with ID understand and design interactions between smart objects. The toolkit adopted a board-game-like format, combining tangible cards and objects to facilitate the creation of simple trigger-action behaviors (e.g., "if button pressed, then light turns on"). Ten participants with ID took part in four workshops, supported by facilitators, where they combined trigger, object, and action cards to ideate meaningful IoT scenarios. This early work highlighted the value of constrained vocabularies, tactile interactions, and collaborative storytelling in fostering understanding and participation.

The second study focused on IoTgoID [8], a tangible, game-based toolkit inspired by the original IoTgo toolkit [10] and redesigned to be accessible to people with ID. IoTgoID supports users in progressing from abstract ideas to concrete IoT prototypes through a modular game board divided into three sequential levels. The toolkit includes action and object cards, 3D-printed replicas of objects and furniture, and a custom-built electronic scanner to combine these cards and 3D replicas into a smart object with real-time IoT behavior. Sessions involve up to four participants and a facilitator collaborating around a game board to co-create functional prototypes. IoTgoID was designed to provide scaffolded learning, tangible manipulation, and playful structure to support engagement, learning, and reflection among participants. The toolkit was designed and validated through 2 workshops that involved 8 participants with ID and one caregiver.

Together, these studies informed a first series of design dimensions for co-design and making toolkits tailored to users with ID, establishing core principles of toolkit affordances, modalities, and interaction. This preliminary design dimension, together with the novel guidelines resulting from the work presented in this paper, are summarized in Fig. 2.

3 Method

This research adopted a user-centered design methodology for the development and evaluation of a novel accessible toolkit built upon guidelines from previous works listed in Sect. 2.1.

This process informs the development of **MakeNodes**, a tangible toolkit that builds from opportunities and limitations observed in COBO and IoTgoID toolkits, shifting the focus from single-device to multi-device prototyping, providing a versatile platform that offers users greater flexibility in ideating and experimenting with customized IoT solutions. The study[1] with MakeNodes was designed to explore aspects of the interaction between users with ID and the toolkit, progressively refining the design based on empirical findings.

The following sections summarize the design, procedure and result of the user study conducted with MakeNodes. A complete technical and methodological description of the toolkit, along with a detailed analysis of the empirical results, can be found in [13].

3.1 *MakeNodes Toolkit*

MakeNodes is a toolkit designed to engage individuals with ID in rapidly creating smart-things networks. The toolkit includes seven devices, called *nodes* (See Fig. 1.A): three sensor nodes (a button, an RFID tag reader, and a motion sensor) and four actuator nodes (a single-color LED light, a multi-color LED light, a buzzer, and a vibration motor). Each sensor node can connect wirelessly with up to four actuator nodes, operating on a trigger/action basis. This connection can be performed by (i) proximity, simply bringing a sensor and actuator node close together to connect them (Fig. 1.B), or (ii) using a scanner, nicknamed the Magic Wand (Fig. 1.C), replicating the interaction modality used in IoTgoID. Built-in magnets and various attachment add-ons enable these nodes to be affixed to diverse object or surface, transforming the room in a smart environment (Fig. 1.D-E).

MakeNodes offers a structured, step-by-step process that starts with pairing sensors and actuators and concludes with deploying the solution within an indoor environment. MakeNodes fosters group collaboration, encouraging participants to reflect and discuss while completing design tasks. Users work together to create a network of sensors and actuators that address specific issues identified within an indoor space.

---

[1] This study received approval from the Ethics Committee of Politecnico di Milano and was conducted with informed consent from participants.

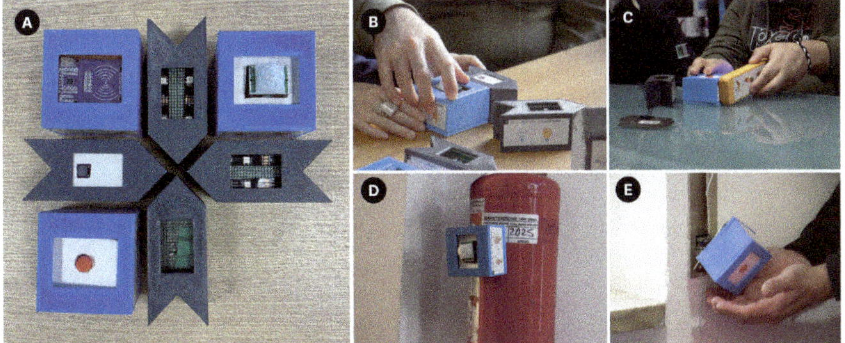

Fig. 1 (A) MakeNodes Toolkit, distinguishes between blue nodes, which serve as sensor nodes, and grey nodes, which function as actuator nodes. (B) Participants connect a sensor (PIR) with an actuator node (Buzzer). (C) A participant employs the smart wand to initiate pairing with a sensor node (button). (D and E) An example of a sensor node deployed in the workshop setting.

3.2 Participants

The study involved 12 participants with ID, comprising five men and seven women aged between 22 and 56. Their IDs ranged from mild to severe (see Table 1). All participants regularly attended a day center located in Milan, Italy. Among the 12 participants, four were part of a micro-community project, which began in July 2011. This project targets women with mild to moderate ID who wish to experience a more autonomous lifestyle. It provides a sheltered living environment where activities related to daily living, social interactions, and continuity with care and education programs are maintained. The involvement of individuals from the micro-community project aimed at investigating the impact of IoT design on improving living conditions in the micro-community's private homes.

3.3 Procedure

Three ninety-minute workshops, each involving four participants, were held in two rooms regularly used by attendees within the facilities of the day center. Both locations featured similar setups, with participants seated around a central table.

The study comprised two phases. During Phase 1, participants engaged in pure co-design activities aimed at investigating if physical affordances could influence the perception of temporal or sequential order, to establish product design guidelines for accessible toolkits. Phase 2 involved practical, hands-on activities using the MakeNodes toolkit. Table 2 outlines the whole structure of the workshops.

Table 1 Data coded for study participants. The letters in the initial column denote the specific workshop each participant attended

Identifier	Gender	YoB	Other information
P1a	F	1982	N/A
P2a	F	1986	N/A
P3a	F	1991	N/A
P4a	F	1968	N/A
P5b	M	2000	Drug-resistant epilepsy, congenital encephalopathy
P6b	M	1997	Emotional regulation disorders, psychosis, and epilepsy
P7b	M	1990	Facial dysmorphism
P8b	M	1987	Alternating phases of space-time disorientation
P9c	F	1991	Mixed disorder of conduct and emotions, drug-resistant epilepsy
P10c	F	1993	Mental impairment, mild Bipolar Affective Disorder
P11c	F	1999	Down Syndrome
P12c	M	1996	N/A

Table 2 A list of tasks for each workshop, categorized by phase

Phase(P)	Task(T)	Task name	Participants	Materials	Duration (minutes)
1	1	Color task	4	20 polystyrene cubes	15
	2	Shape task	4	20 cardboard shapes	15
2	3	Embodied interaction	4	MakeNodes toolkit	20
	4	Naturalistic observation	4 divided in 2 sub-groups	MakeNodes toolkit	40

4 Key Results and Emerging Themes

All participants engaged collaboratively in groups to ideate and design meaningful node networks. Despite encountering varying levels of challenge, each group completed the tasks with only verbal prompts provided by the researcher. In total, participants developed 12 distinct node networks designed to enhance the shared spaces of the day center and to address issues related to peer safety and social interaction. The toolkit activities effectively addressed common barriers to IoT comprehension, such as understanding trigger-action relationships and basic connection models. It is important to acknowledge that individuals with ID exhibit a wide range of autonomy and interpersonal skills, even when possessing similar IQ levels. This heterogeneity complicates the generalization of findings to broader populations. Nonetheless, the results from MakeNodes demonstrate that a selected group was capable of co-designing practical solutions that reflected the resources available at the center and the participants' contextual needs. A series of themes emerges from the results:

Impact of Real-World Relevance The context for which participants were required to design significantly influenced their ideation capabilities. Individuals designing solutions for environments they personally managed (e.g., their shared apartment, in the case of the participant from the micro-community project) generated more context-aware and initiative-driven ideas than those working in shared or less personally significant spaces. This highlights the importance of perceived responsibility and emotional connection to the design context in fostering meaningful participation.

Accessibility Through Physical Affordances Participants responded well to the physical affordances embedded in MakeNodes. Color and shape combinations show positive results in helping convey functional roles (sensor vs. actuator), and immediate feedback from the nodes (e.g., lights or sounds) enhanced comprehension. However, while shapes and colors supported understanding of individual components, they were less effective at conveying more abstract concepts like temporal sequencing. This suggests the need for multi-modal scaffolding, combining visual, tactile, and feedback-based cues.

Usability of Pairing Interactions Both proximity-based and wand-based pairing methods were usable by all participants. While proximity pairing was more intuitive, the Magic Wand, despite an initial learning curve, was preferred by many due to its novelty and sensory feedback. This indicates that user engagement can outweigh strict ease-of-use in some contexts, and both methods serve complementary roles in sustaining interest and accommodating different preferences.

Embodied Exploration and Instruction Embodied exploration alone was insufficient for users to fully grasp all toolkit interactions without facilitator support. The printed instructions on each node needed to be supplemented by guided demonstrations. Nevertheless, once explained, participants exhibited strong retention and effective use of the toolkit. This suggests that combining initial guided practice with intuitive feedback mechanisms offers the best path toward independent use.

Long-Term Usability and Caregiver Support MakeNodes was designed for post-study sustainability, enabling caregivers to continue using the toolkit without technical support. Rechargeable batteries, simplified components, and minimal setup requirements made it feasible for day-to-day application. Future iterations could enhance autonomy further by integrating magnetic chargers and high-capacity batteries, streamlining maintenance for caregivers, and extending usage in diverse environments.

Adaptability Across Contexts Unlike earlier toolkits that required context-specific customization, MakeNodes supports general-purpose adaptability. Its node-based system operates independently of specific physical contexts, reducing the need for scenario-specific assets. This flexibility allows it to be reused across different user groups and locations, increasing its potential for broader application and dissemination beyond the original research setting.

5 Design Guidelines for Accessible Making Toolkits

The insights and results from the study with MakeNodes, combined with the preliminary results from previous works (See Sect. 2.1), drive the definition of a comprehensive set of interaction and design guidelines that can guide the design of futures

---

Design Guidelines for Accessible Making Toolkits for ID

FROM PREVIOUS STUDIES

Easy-to-Manipulate
Toolkits should feature large surfaces and easily manipulable materials and connectors.

Esnure Balanced Roles
If role are assigned, they must be balanced to match the competencies of participants. Roles should be aligned with individual skills and preferences to enhance engagement.

Promote screenless interactions
Literature highlights the importance of multimodal guidance to ensure the inclusion of diverse participants and to utilize various skill sets. Implementing a conversational assistant could address this requirement without needing a screen, thereby avoiding additional stimuli that may distract and hinder social interactions.

Scaffolding the experience
If present, toolkits should exhibit a linear progression across different levels. Such progression enabled participants to achieve small successes and develop a sense of competence.

Reflections and Revisions sessions
Toolkits should ensure an immediate connection between reflective stimuli and necessary revisions. Additionally, discussions sessions should be concise to facilitate small wins during dialogues and overall gameplay

Recall Real-world Objects
Reflections become easier when participants could relate to real physical objects they had or can interact with.

Materialize concepts
Abstract concepts need to be materialized for better comprehension. For example, arrows guided individuals through prototyping tasks, cards represented key components and design choices or concretized abstract concepts like states of input and output.

Role of Self-Exploration
Encouraging self-exploration of toolkit elements and features can promote independence and personal agency. This approach leverages participants' inherent curiosity.

Conversational Assistants
According to existing research, conversational assistants have the potential to provide additional support to individuals with ID when used in conjunction with a caregiver. Furthermore, a conversational assistant could mitigate the need for a moderator.

Define clear and scaffolded goals
Toolkits could benefit from distinctly separating goals according to each level and player, aligned with distinct player roles, such as game master, speaker, or those responsible for stimulating reflections.

Balance the Number of Choices
Literature recommends allowing room for free choices and exploration. However, the number of choices must be balanced and suitable for participants' decision-making abilities.

FROM MAKENODES STUDY

Promote long-term sustainabiltity
Designing adaptable, reusable components that are cost-effective and easy to implement, ensure long-term sustainability, particularly important in educational settings where resources are often limited. Design to be highly versatile, with the ability to adapt to new learning contexts and making it easier for caregivers and educators to implement the toolkit, further extending its impact.

Provide multi-modal cues
Using visual cues alone can be insufficient to support user understanding, in this case an initial guided practice can be paired with visual, tactile, and feedback-based cues to offers the best path toward independent use.

Focus on Real-world, familiar scenarios
A sense of responsibility and emotional connection to the design context can fostered participation. Incorporating real-world contexts in the design activities enhanced the relevance and applicability of the tasks participants performed.

Encourage hands-on activities
Hands-on activities foster greater engagement than unstructured reflection.

Enure Flexibility in Social Interaction
While structured interactions are beneficial in reducing confusion, flexibility in social interactions can aid in task success and reflective activities, offering a balance between guidance and autonomy.

Encourage Autonomy and Self-exploration
Minimizing instructions can encourage participants to take ownership of their learning process. The immediate feedback provided by the toolkit also supported understanding without the need for extensive guidance, promoting autonomy.

Fig. 2 Guidelines from previous studies (white background) are integrated with new insights from user studies with MakeNodes (grey background)

making toolkits for people with ID. Figure 2 organizes the complete set of guidelines in the form of a design manifesto for accessible making toolkits for people with ID.

6 Conclusion

The MakeNodes toolkit successfully engaged adults with ID in IoT network design. All participants actively contributed to creating meaningful networks of smart devices tailored to everyday challenges, showing meaningful collaboration and sustained interest. Despite individual differences in autonomy and communication abilities, the majority successfully understood key concepts such as trigger-action logic and connection modalities.

Building on lessons learned from previous work, the study with MakeNodes provided empirical evidence that with appropriate design and interaction features, a making toolkit can be designed to be accessible for people with ID, establishing a step towards accessibility. For practitioners and researchers, these findings should encourage to design phygital tools and interfaces that integrate physical interaction with digital functionality, thereby democratizing IoT prototyping. The demonstrated success of the tangible approach in this study supports its broader applicability. HCI researchers could build on defined guidelines to develop or adapt similar tangible toolkits for other domains, such as home automation or robotics, with the aim of including individuals with ID in a wider range of technology design activities.

References

1. D. Chapko, P. Frumiento, N. Edwards, L. Emeh, D. Kennedy, D. McNicholas, M. Overton, M. Snead, R. Steward, J.M. Sutton, E. Jeffreys, C. Long, J. Croll-Knight, B. Connors, S. Castell-Ward, D. Coke, B. McPeake, W. Renel, C. McGinley, A. Remington, D. Whittuck, J. Kieffer, S. Ewans, M. Williams, M. Grierson, we have been magnified for years—now you are under the microscope!: co-researchers with learning disabilities created an online survey to challenge public understanding of learning disabilities, in *Proceedings of the 2020 CHI Conference on Human Factors in Computing Systems*, CHI '20, New York, NY, USA (Association for Computing Machinery 2020), pp. 1–17
2. G. Cosentino, D. Morra, M. Gelsomini, M. Matera, M. Mores, Cobo: a card-based toolkit for co-designing smart outdoor experiences with people with intellectual disability, in *IFIP Conference on Human-Computer Interaction* (Springer, 2021), pp. 149–169
3. K. Ellis, E. Dao, O. Smith, S. Lindsay, P. Olivier, Tapeblocks: a making toolkit for people living with intellectual disabilities, in *Proceedings of the 2021 CHI Conference on Human Factors in Computing Systems*, CHI '21, New York, NY, USA (Association for Computing Machinery, 2021)
4. G. Ermacora, M.L. Lupetti, L. Pei, Design for all. l making and learning for and with people with disabilities, in *Proceedings of the 12th International Conference on Education Technology and Computers*, ICETC '20, New York, NY, USA (Association for Computing Machinery, 2021), pp. 41–45

5. T.P. Falcão, Action-effect mappings in tangible interaction for children with intellectual disabilities. Int. J. Learn. Technol. **12**(4), 294–314 (2017)
6. A. Gaggioli, Phygital spaces: when atoms meet bits. Cyberpsychol. Behav. Soc. Netw. **20**(12), 774–774 (2017). (PMID: 29243961)
7. M. Gelsomini, M. Spitale, F. Garzotto, Phygital interfaces for people with intellectual disability: an exploratory study at a social care center. Multimedia Tools Appl. **80**(26–27), 34843–34874 (2021)
8. R. Gennari, M. Matera, A. Melonio, M. Mores, D. Morra, M. Rizvi, A rapid-prototyping toolkit for people with intellectual disabilities. Int. J. Hum.-Comput. Stud. **192**, 103347 (2024)
9. R. Gennari, M. Matera, D. Morra, A. Melonio, M. Rizvi, Design for social digital well-being with young generations: engage them and make them reflect. Int. J. Hum.-Comput. Stud. **173**, 103006 (2023)
10. R. Gennari, M. Matera, D. Morra, A. Melonio, M. Rizvi, Design for social digital well-being with young generations: Engage them and make them reflect. Int. J. Hum.-Comput. Stud. **173**, 103006 (2023)
11. J.A. Kientz, M.S. Goodwin, G.R. Hayes, G.D. Abowd, *Interactive Technologies for Autism*, 1st ed. (Morgan and Claypool Publishers, 2013)
12. L. Martin, The promise of the maker movement for education. J. Pre-College Eng. Edu. Res. (J-PEER) **5** (2015)
13. D. Morra, G. Caslini, M. Mores, F. Garzotto, M. Matera, Makenodes: opening connected-iot making to people with intellectual disability. Int. J. Hum.-Comput. Stud. **190**, 103325 (2024)
14. N. Robb, B. Boyle, Y. Politis, N. Newbutt, H.J. Kuo, C. Sung, Participatory technology design for autism and cognitive disabilities: a narrative overview of issues and techniques, in *Recent Advances in Technologies for Inclusive Well-Being: Virtual Patients, Gamification and Simulation*, pp. 469–485 (2021)
15. H. Senaratne, S. Ananthanarayan, K. Ellis, Tronicboards: an accessible electronics toolkit for people with intellectual disabilities, in *Proceedings of the 2022 CHI Conference on Human Factors in Computing Systems*, CHI '22, New York, NY, USA (Association for Computing Machinery, 2022)

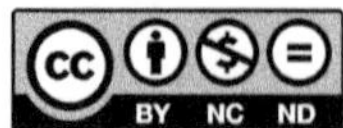

Multi-armed Bandits Algorithms for Pricing and Advertising

Marco Mussi

Abstract Nowadays, when it comes to selling a product online, two of the most significant factors are the pricing strategy and the investments in advertising. When determining the price of a product, it is essential to strike a balance. The price should neither be set too low, as this would result in a reduced revenue, nor too high, as it may deter potential buyers. The amount of money we invest in advertising should be balanced to let people know our offer without overspending. These two aspects are usually handled disjointedly by humans, but this may lead to suboptimal solutions. In this work, we focus on the adoption of online learning algorithms to solve the task of finding the optimal price for a product and understand how to advertise it properly. We face various aspects of pricing and advertising, offering theoretical frameworks to address the associated challenges. We start discussing pricing methods, with emphasis on the problem of learning in the presence of temporal dynamics. Then, we discuss the theoretical aspects of advertising, with a particular focus on marketing mix models. Finally, we bring together the problems of pricing and advertising, presenting a unified view.

1 Introduction

Motivated by the rapid increase in the quantity of data and the exponential growth of online platforms, companies are continually seeking innovative strategies to enhance their market presence, capture consumer attention, and optimize their pricing models. Machine Learning (ML) has emerged in recent years as a groundbreaking transformative force, empowering organizations to revolutionize the way they price products and promote them through advertising. The traditional paradigms of pricing and advertising, once reliant on static models and generalized strategies, are rapidly giving way to data-driven, adaptive approaches powered by ML algorithms.

M. Mussi (✉)
Politecnico di Milano, Piazza Leonardo da Vinci 32, Milan, Italy
e-mail: marco.mussi@polimi.it

C. Cappiello (ed.), *Special Topics in Information Technology*,
PoliMI SpringerBriefs, https://doi.org/10.1007/978-3-032-12359-6_3

In this work, we face the problem of online decision-making in the context of dynamic pricing and advertising budget optimization. These two topics are, indeed, two sides of the same coin. In order to sell a product, we must be able to select both a price that is proper for the reference market and advertise it properly. The price should neither be set too low, as this would result in reduced revenue from the single sale, nor too high, as it may deter potential buyers. The amount of money we invest in advertising should be balanced to let people know of us without overspending and reaching people who are not interested. The goal, indeed, is to optimize the combination of pricing and advertising policies to increase our revenue.

Structure and Contributions. In Sect. 2, we formulate a new approach [1] for handling dynamic pricing using Multi-Armed Bandits (MABs, [2]) methods taking into account the temporal dependencies through the introduction of AutoRegressive (AR) processes to model such a dependency. Such processes are useful to represent trends that are not captured by standard MABs. In Sect. 3, we focus on the problem of budget optimization in online advertising, and in particular, on the problem of budget optimization in Marketing Mix Models (MMMs). We propose [3], a framework to face the problem of optimizing the budget allocation in MMMs online. In Sect. 4, we face the problem of jointly optimizing the price at which we want to sell an item and the expenditure to advertise it. We propose [4, 5], a new framework for handling the problem in which the reward is factored and observable in intermediate steps, and we design an algorithm to solve this problem with theoretical guarantees.[1] These three parts are all binded each other from (i) the scope of the proposed algorithms, whose final goal in all the cases is to improve the revenues due to the sales we perform, and (ii) the methodology used to pursue the goal, as all the algorithms presented in this work are based on MABs.

2 Dynamic Pricing

In this section, we consider the problem of finding the optimal price for a given product. Our goal is to maximize a certain index, e.g., volumes, turnover, or profit. Usually, pricing algorithms focus on the *one-step* performance [7]. These solutions, however, fail in modeling the *long-term* phenomena that a pricing strategy inherently presents. Indeed, with one-step solutions, we fail (i) to model the long-term effect such as customer loyalty, and (ii) to capture the different demands of loyal and non-loyal customers. This problem, even if ubiquitous in the real world, is unexplored in the literature, as existing approaches struggle to correctly deal with these autoregressive dynamics. Motivated by the problem described above, we propose a novel setting, named *AutoRegressive Bandits* (ARBs), in which the reward follows an AR process of order n whose parameters depend on the actions.

---

[1] For all the formal proofs and additional results, we refer the interested reader to the works cited above and to [6].

2.1 Setting

Let $T \in \mathbb{N}$ be the learning horizon. At every round $t \in [\![T]\!]$, the learner chooses an action $a_t \in \mathcal{A} := [\![k]\!]$, among the $k \in \mathbb{N}$ available ones. In the ARB setting, the reward evolves according to an *autoregressive process of order n* (AR(n)). Thus, the learner observes a noisy reward x_t of the form:

$$ x_t = \gamma_0(a_t) + \sum_{i=1}^{n} \gamma_i(a_t) x_{t-i} + \epsilon_t, $$

where $\gamma_0(a_t) \in \mathbb{R}$ and $(\gamma_i(a_t))_{i \in [\![n]\!]} \in \mathbb{R}^n$ are the unknown *parameters* depending on chosen action a_t, and ϵ_t is σ^2-subgaussian noise. The reward evolution can be also expressed as $x_t = \langle \boldsymbol{\gamma}(a_t), \mathbf{z}_{t-1} \rangle + \epsilon_t$, where $\mathbf{z}_{t-1} := (1, x_{t-1}, \dots, x_{t-n})^{\mathrm{T}} \in \mathcal{Z} := \{1\} \times \mathcal{X}^n$ is the *vector of past rewards* expressing past history, and $\boldsymbol{\gamma}(a) := (\gamma_0(a), \dots, \gamma_n(a))^{\mathrm{T}} \in \mathbb{R}^{n+1}$ is the *parameter vector*, defined for every $a \in \mathcal{A}$. We introduce the following assumptions:

a. (Non-negative coefficients) $\gamma_i(a) \geq 0$ for every $a \in \mathcal{A}, i \in [\![0, n]\!]$;
b. (Stability) $\Gamma := \max_{a \in \mathcal{A}} \sum_{i=1}^{n} \gamma_i(a) < 1$;
c. (Boundedness) $m := \max_{a \in \mathcal{A}} \gamma_0(a) < +\infty$.

The performance of a policy π is evaluated in terms of the *expected cumulative reward* over the horizon T, defined as:

$$ J(\pi, T) := \mathbb{E}\left[\sum_{t=1}^{T} x_t \right]. $$

A policy π^* is *optimal* if it maximizes the expected average reward, i.e., $\pi^* \in \arg\max_\pi J(\pi, T)$. The goal of the learner is to minimize the *expected cumulative (policy) regret* by playing a policy π, competing against the optimal policy π^* over the *learning horizon T*:

$$ R(\pi, T) = J(\pi^*, T) - J(\pi, T) = \mathbb{E}\left[\sum_{t=1}^{T} r_t \right], $$

where $r_t := x_t^* - x_t$ is the instantaneous policy regret and $(x_t^*)_{t \in [\![T]\!]}$ is the sequence of rewards observed by playing the optimal policy. The optimal policy, which maximizes the expected cumulative reward, is $\pi_t^* \in \arg\max_{a \in \mathcal{A}} \langle \boldsymbol{\gamma}(a), \mathbf{z}_{t-1} \rangle$.

Mapping to Pricing. The pricing problem discussed above can be mapped to the ARB setting. Imagine we want to maximize the volumes over time. The volumes are our reward x_t, and the history of our rewards $x_{t-1}, \dots, x_{t-n}$ provides an indication of the loyal customer pool over the past n units of time (e.g., weeks). The ARB setting allows modeling a reward which is the contribution of both new customers (via γ_0) and the loyal customer pool (via $\gamma_1, \dots, \gamma_n$). Specifically, the price (our *action*),

26   M. Mussi

Input: Regularization param. λ, AR order n, Exploration coefficients $(\beta_{t-1})_{t\in[\![T]\!]}$
Initialize $\mathbf{V}_0(a) = \lambda\mathbf{I}_{n+1}$, $\mathbf{b}_0(a) = \mathbf{0}_{n+1}$, $\widehat{\boldsymbol{\gamma}}_0(a) = \mathbf{0}_{n+1}$, $\forall a \in \mathcal{A}$, $\mathbf{z}_0 = (1, 0, \ldots, 0)^{\mathrm{T}}$, $t \leftarrow 1$
for $t \in [\![T]\!]$ **do**
$\quad$ Compute $a_t \in \arg\max_{a\in\mathcal{A}} \mathrm{UCB}_t(a) := \langle\widehat{\boldsymbol{\gamma}}_{t-1}(a), \mathbf{z}_{t-1}\rangle + \beta_{t-1}(a)\,\|\mathbf{z}_{t-1}\|_{\mathbf{V}_{t-1}(a)^{-1}}$
$\quad$ Play action a_t and observe $x_t = \langle\boldsymbol{\gamma}(a_t), \mathbf{z}_{t-1}\rangle + \epsilon_t$
$\quad$ Update $\forall a \in \mathcal{A}$:
$\qquad \mathbf{V}_t(a) = \mathbf{V}_{t-1}(a) + \mathbf{z}_{t-1}\mathbf{z}_{t-1}^{\mathrm{T}}\,\mathbb{1}_{\{a=a_t\}}$
$\qquad \mathbf{b}_t(a) = \mathbf{b}_{t-1}(a) + \mathbf{z}_{t-1}x_t\,\mathbb{1}_{\{a=a_t\}}$
$\qquad \widehat{\boldsymbol{\gamma}}_t(a) = \mathbf{V}_t(a)^{-1}\mathbf{b}_t(a)$
$\quad$ Update $\mathbf{z}_t = (1, x_t, \ldots, x_{t-n+1})^{\mathrm{T}}$, $\quad t \leftarrow t+1$
end

$$\textbf{Algorithm 1: } \texttt{AR-UCB}.$$

induces different values of the coefficient $\boldsymbol{\gamma}(a_t)$, to represent the different demand curves that loyal and new customers might have.

2.2 Algorithm

We present AutoRegressive Upper Confidence Bound (AR-UCB, Algorithm 1), an optimistic regret minimization algorithm for the ARB setting. AR-UCB leverages the myopic optimal policy for ARBs and implements an incremental regularized least squares procedure to estimate the unknown parameters $\boldsymbol{\gamma}(a)$, for every action $a \in \mathcal{A}$ independently. The algorithm requires knowledge of the order n of the AR process, although this knowledge can be replaced with that of an upper bound $\bar{n} > n$ of the AR order. AR-UCB starts by initializing for all the actions $a \in \mathcal{A}$ the Gram matrix $\mathbf{V}_0(a) = \lambda\mathbf{I}_{n+1}$, where $\lambda > 0$ is the Ridge regularization parameter, the vectors $\mathbf{b}_0(a) = \widehat{\boldsymbol{\gamma}}_0(a) = \mathbf{0}_{n+1}$, and the observations vector $\mathbf{z}_0 = (1, 0, \ldots, 0)^{\mathrm{T}}$. Then, for each round $t \in [\![T]\!]$, AR-UCB computes the *Upper Confidence Bound* (UCB) index for every $a \in \mathcal{A}$ and select the optimistic action a_t as:

$$a_t \in \underset{a\in\mathcal{A}}{\arg\max}\ \mathrm{UCB}_t(a) := \langle\widehat{\boldsymbol{\gamma}}_{t-1}(a), \mathbf{z}_{t-1}\rangle + \beta_{t-1}(a)\,\|\mathbf{z}_{t-1}\|_{\mathbf{V}_{t-1}(a)^{-1}}\,,$$

where $\widehat{\boldsymbol{\gamma}}_{t-1}(a)$ is the most recent estimate of the parameter vector $\boldsymbol{\gamma}(a)$, $\mathbf{z}_{t-1} = (1, x_{t-1}, \ldots, x_{t-n})^{\mathrm{T}}$ is the observations vector, and $\beta_{t-1}(a) > 0$ is a properly selected exploration coefficient. The index $\mathrm{UCB}_t(a)$ is designed to be optimistic, i.e., $\langle\boldsymbol{\gamma}(a), \mathbf{z}_{t-1}\rangle \leq \mathrm{UCB}_t(a)$ with high probability for all $a \in \mathcal{A}$. Then, action a_t is executed and the new reward x_t is observed. This sample is employed to update the Gram matrix estimate $\mathbf{V}_t(a_t)$, the vector $\mathbf{b}_t(a_t)$, and the estimate $\widehat{\boldsymbol{\gamma}}_t(a_t)$.

Regret Guarantees. `AR-UCB` suffers an expected policy regret as follows:

$$\mathbb{E}[R(\text{AR-UCB}, T)] \leq \tilde{O}\left(\frac{(m+\sigma)(n+1)^{3/2}\sqrt{kT}}{(1-\Gamma)^2}\right).$$

3 Advertising Optimization

In online advertising, the process that leads to a *conversion* presents complex dynamics and may involve different types of campaigns, and a profitable budget investment policy has to account for their interplay [8]. Indeed, a conversion should be attributed not only to the latest ad and the *joint* consideration of campaigns is fundamental. Consider a simplified model with two types of campaigns: *awareness* (i.e., impression) ads and *conversion* ads. If we evaluate our performance in terms of conversions, we observe that impression ads are not effective, so we will be tempted to reduce their budget. However, this approach may be sub-optimal, as impression ads enhance the effectiveness of conversion ads by increasing the likelihood that users will convert. In addition, the effect of some ads, especially the ones via television, may be delayed, and it has been demonstrated [9] that users remember ads in a vanishing way. To model this scenario, we propose *Dynamical Linear Bandits* (DLBs), to model these effects as a linear system with hidden state.

3.1 Setting

In a DLB, we have a *hidden* state $\mathbf{x} \in \mathcal{X}$, where $\mathcal{X} \subseteq \mathbb{R}^n$ is the state space. At each round t, the environment is in the hidden state $\mathbf{x}_t \in \mathcal{X}$, the learner chooses an action $\mathbf{u}_t \in \mathcal{U}$, where $\mathcal{U} \subseteq \mathbb{R}^d$ is the action space. The learner receives a noisy reward $y_t = \langle \boldsymbol{\omega}, \mathbf{x}_t \rangle + \langle \boldsymbol{\theta}, \mathbf{u}_t \rangle + \eta_t$, where $\boldsymbol{\omega} \in \mathbb{R}^n, \boldsymbol{\theta} \in \mathbb{R}^d$ are unknown, and η_t is σ^2-subgaussian noise. Then, the environment evolves according to the unknown linear dynamics $\mathbf{x}_{t+1} = \mathbf{A}\mathbf{x}_t + \mathbf{B}\mathbf{u}_t + \boldsymbol{\epsilon}_t$, where $\mathbf{A} \in \mathbb{R}^{n \times n}$ is the dynamic matrix, $\mathbf{B} \in \mathbb{R}^{n \times d}$ is the action-state matrix, and $\boldsymbol{\epsilon}_t$ is a σ^2-subgaussian noise vector. We consider stable systems in which $\mathbf{A}$ has maximum eigenvalues smaller than 1 in module ($\rho(\mathbf{A}) < 1$). Given a policy π, we define its *(infinite-horizon) expected average reward*:

$$J(\pi) := \liminf_{H \to +\infty} \mathbb{E}\left[\frac{1}{H}\sum_{t=1}^{H} y_t\right].$$

A policy π^* is an *optimal policy* if it maximizes the expected average reward. We evaluate policies in terms of *expected cumulative regret*, i.e., the sum over time of the difference in performance w.r.t. the optimal policy π^*.

Input: Regularization param. λ, Exploration coeffs. $(\beta_{t-1})_{t \in [\![T]\!]}$, Spectral radius UB $\overline{\rho}$
Initialize $t \leftarrow 1$, $\mathbf{V}_0 = \lambda \mathbf{I}_d$, $\mathbf{b}_0 = \mathbf{0}_d$, $\widehat{\mathbf{h}}_0 = \mathbf{0}_d$
Define $M = \min\{M' \in \mathbb{N} : \sum_{m=1}^{M'} 1 + \lfloor \frac{\log m}{\log(1/\overline{\rho})} \rfloor > T\} - 1$
for $m \in [\![M]\!]$ **do**
     Compute $\mathbf{u}_t \in \arg\max_{\mathbf{u} \in \mathcal{U}} \text{UCB}_t(\mathbf{u})$ where $\text{UCB}_t(\mathbf{u}) := \langle \widehat{\mathbf{h}}_{t-1}, \mathbf{u} \rangle + \beta_{t-1} \|\mathbf{u}\|_{\mathbf{V}_{t-1}^{-1}}$
     Play arm $\mathbf{u}_t$ and observe reward y_t
     Define $H_m = \lfloor \frac{\log m}{\log(1/\overline{\rho})} \rfloor$
     for $j \in [\![H_m]\!]$ **do**
         Play arm $\mathbf{u}_t = \mathbf{u}_{t-1}$ and observe y_t
         Update $\mathbf{V}_t = \mathbf{V}_{t-1}$, $\mathbf{b}_t = \mathbf{b}_{t-1}$, $t \leftarrow t+1$
     end
     Update and compute: $\mathbf{V}_t = \mathbf{V}_{t-1} + \mathbf{u}_t \mathbf{u}_t^{\mathrm{T}}$, $\mathbf{b}_t = \mathbf{b}_{t-1} + \mathbf{u}_t y_t$, $\widehat{\mathbf{h}}_t = \mathbf{V}_t^{-1} \mathbf{b}_t$, $t \leftarrow t+1$
end

Algorithm 2: `DynLin-UCB`.

Lower Bound. We characterize the expected regret that every policy π will suffer:

$$\mathbb{E}[R(\pi, T)] \geq \Omega \left(\frac{d\sqrt{T}}{\sqrt{(1 - \rho(\mathbf{A}))}} \right).$$

Mapping to Advertising. Budget allocation in MMMs can be mapped to a DLB where the budget is our action $\mathbf{u}_t$, the value of awareness (not measurable) is the hidden state $\mathbf{x}_t$, and the reward y_t is the number of conversions (observed).

3.2 Algorithm

We present an *optimistic* regret minimization algorithm for the DLBs setting. Dynamical Linear Upper Confidence Bound (`DynLin-UCB`, Algorithm 2) requires the knowledge of an upper-bound $\overline{\rho} < 1$ on the spectral radius of $\mathbf{A}$. To assess the quality of action $\mathbf{u} \in \mathcal{U}$, we *persist* in applying it so that the system approximately reaches the corresponding steady state and, then, observe the reward y_t, representing a reliable estimate of $J(\mathbf{u}) = \langle \mathbf{h}, \mathbf{u} \rangle$, where $\mathbf{h} = \theta + \mathbf{B}^{\mathrm{T}} (\mathbf{I}_n - \mathbf{A})^{-\mathrm{T}} \omega$ is what we call a *Markovian* vector representing the whole system at the steady state. We shall show that the number of rounds needed to approximately reach such a steady state is logarithmic in the learning horizon T and depends on $\overline{\rho}$. `DynLin-UCB` subdivides the learning horizon T into M *epochs*. Each epoch $m \in [\![M]\!]$ is composed of $H_m + 1$ rounds, where $H_m = \lfloor \log m / \log(1/\overline{\rho}) \rfloor$. At the beginning of each epoch, `DynLin-UCB` computes the UCB index defined for every $\mathbf{u} \in \mathcal{U}$ as $\text{UCB}_t(\mathbf{u}) := \langle \widehat{\mathbf{h}}_{t-1}, \mathbf{u} \rangle + \beta_{t-1} \|\mathbf{u}\|_{\mathbf{V}_{t-1}^{-1}}$, where $\widehat{\mathbf{h}}_{t-1} = \mathbf{V}_{t-1}^{-1} \mathbf{b}_{t-1}$ is the Ridge regression estimator of Markov parameter $\mathbf{h}$, and $\beta_{t-1} > 0$ is a properly selected exploration coefficient. Similar to `Lin-UCB` [10], the index $\text{UCB}_t(\mathbf{u})$ is designed to be optimistic, i.e., $J(\mathbf{u}) \leq \text{UCB}_t(\mathbf{u})$ in high-probability for all $\mathbf{u} \in \mathcal{U}$. The optimistic action $\mathbf{u}_t \in \arg\max_{\mathbf{u} \in \mathcal{U}} \text{UCB}_t(\mathbf{u})$ is executed and persisted for the next H_m rounds. In this way, at the end of each epoch, the reward y_t is an almost-unbiased sample of the steady-state performance $J(\mathbf{u}_t)$, which can be employed to update the $\mathbf{V}_t$ and $\mathbf{b}_t$.

Regret Guarantees. Considering a proper selection of β_t and the knowledge of the upper bounds $\overline{\rho} < 1$, DynLin-UCB suffers an expected regret bounded as:

$$\mathbb{E}[R(\texttt{DynLin-UCB}, T)] \leq \tilde{O}\left(\frac{d\sqrt{T}}{1-\overline{\rho}} + \frac{\sqrt{dT}}{(1-\overline{\rho})^{3/2}} + \frac{1}{(1-\rho(\mathbf{A}))^2}\right).$$

4 Joint Pricing and Advertising

In this section, we present a model for jointly optimizing pricing and advertising. We have to coherently choose (i) the *price* and (ii) how much *budget* to invest in advertising. The price we set determines the willingness of the users to buy a given item, i.e., the *conversion rate*, while the advertising budget influences the number of people that will see an item, i.e., the number of *impressions*. At every step, we select a *price-budget* couple, and we observe the *conversion rate*, which depends on the price, and the number of *impressions*, which depends on the *budget* we invest in advertising. This scenario can be treated as a standard MAB by looking just at the reward (i.e., the revenue) and considering price-budget couples as actions. However, this solution is very inefficient, and the resulting problem will present an unnecessarily large action space, including all the possible combinations of actions. Given that, we now propose a general model, called *Factored Reward Bandits* (FRBs), able to characterize the problem of optimizing this scenario.

4.1 Setting

Let $T \in \mathbb{N}$ be the time horizon. In a FRB, at every round $t \in [\![T]\!]$ we choose an action vector $\mathbf{a}(t) = (a_1(t), \ldots, a_d(t))$ in a given action space $\mathcal{A} := [\![k_1]\!] \times \cdots \times [\![k_d]\!]$, where $k_i \in \mathbb{N}$ is the number of options for the ith action component, and $d \in \mathbb{N}$ is the action vector dimension (i.e., the number of components that the learner must select). As a result, we observe a vector of d components $\mathbf{x}(t) = (x_1(t), \ldots, x_d(t))$. The ith component $x_i(t)$ of the observation vector $\mathbf{x}(t)$ is the effect of the ith action component $a_i(t)$ in the action vector $\mathbf{a}(t)$. Every component of the observation vector $\mathbf{x}(t)$ is independent of the others and sampled from a distribution $x_i(t) \sim \nu_{i,a_i(t)}$. We consider stochastic observations, i.e., $x_i(t) = \mu_{i,a_i(t)} + \epsilon_i(t)$, where $\mu_{i,a_i(t)}$ is the expected value of the observation of action a_i of the ith component, and $\epsilon_i(t)$ is σ^2-subgaussian noise. We consider bounded expected values for the observations, i.e., $\mu_{i,a_i} \in [0, 1]$ for every $i \in [\![d]\!]$, $a_i \in [\![k_i]\!]$. The reward is given by the product of the observations $r(t) = \prod_{i \in [\![d]\!]} x_i(t)$. In the FRB setting, the optimal action is:

Input: Exploration param. α, Subgaussianity proxy σ, Action space dim. k_i, $\forall i \in [\![d]\!]$
Initialize $\forall a_i \in [\![k_i]\!]$, $i \in [\![d]\!]$: $\quad N_{i,a_i}(0) \leftarrow 0$, $\widehat{\mu}_{i,a_i}(0) \leftarrow 0$
for $t \in [\![T]\!]$ **do**
$\quad$ Select $\mathbf{a}(t) \in \arg\max_{\mathbf{a}=(a_1,\ldots a_d) \in \mathcal{A}} \prod_{i \in [\![d]\!]} \mathrm{UCB}_{i,a_i}(t)$
$\quad$ Play $\mathbf{a}(t)$ and observe $\mathbf{x}(t) = (x_1(t), \ldots, x_d(t))$
$\quad$ Update $\forall i \in [\![d]\!]$:
$\qquad \widehat{\mu}_{i,a_i(t)}(t) \leftarrow \frac{\widehat{\mu}_{i,a_i(t)}(t-1) \, N_{i,a_i(t)}(t-1)+x_i(t)}{N_{i,a_i(t)}(t-1)+1}$, $\quad N_{i,a_i(t)}(t) \leftarrow N_{i,a_i(t)}(t-1)+1$
$\quad$ Update $\forall i \in [\![d]\!], \forall j \in [\![k_i]\!] \setminus \{a_i(t)\}$: $\widehat{\mu}_{i,j}(t) \leftarrow \widehat{\mu}_{i,j}(t-1)$, $N_{i,j}(t) \leftarrow N_{i,j}(t-1)$
end

Algorithm 3: F-UCB.

$$\mathbf{a}^* = (a_1^*, \ldots, a_d^*) \in \arg\max_{\mathbf{a}=(a_1,\ldots,a_d) \in \mathcal{A}} \prod_{i \in [\![d]\!]} \mu_{i,a_i},$$

and we can factorize the learning problem observing that $a_i^* \in \arg\max_{a_i \in [\![k_i]\!]} \mu_{i,a_i}$ for every $i \in [\![d]\!]$. We call $\mu_i^* = \mu_{i,a_i^*}$ the expected value of the optimal action of the ith component. Given a policy π, we define its *cumulative regret* as:

$$R(\pi, T) := T \prod_{i \in [\![d]\!]} \mu_i^* - \sum_{t \in [\![T]\!]} \prod_{i \in [\![d]\!]} \mu_{i,a_i(t)}.$$

The goal of the learner is to minimize the *expected cumulative regret* $\mathbb{E}[R(\pi, T)]$.

Lower Bound. We characterize the expected regret that every policy π will suffer:

$$\mathbb{E}[R(\pi, T)] \geq \Omega\left(\sqrt{T \sum_{i \in [\![d]\!]} k_i}\right).$$

4.2 Algorithm

We present an *optimistic* regret minimization algorithm for the FRB setting. Factored Upper Confidence Bound (F-UCB, Algorithm 3) is inspired by the optimistic bound of UCB1 [11, 12]. The algorithm requires as input the action space dimension k_i for every $i \in [\![d]\!]$, the exploration parameter α, and the subgaussianity coefficient σ. For every round $t \in [\![T]\!]$, we estimate the best optimistic action, i.e., the action $\mathbf{a}(t)$ maximizing the index:

$$\mathbf{a}(t) \in \arg\max_{\mathbf{a}=(a_1,\ldots,a_d) \in \mathcal{A}} \prod_{i \in [\![d]\!]} \mathrm{UCB}_{i,a_i}(t),$$

where $\mathrm{UCB}_{i,a_i}(t) := \widehat{\mu}_{i,a_i}(t-1) + \sigma\sqrt{\frac{\alpha \log t}{N_{i,a_i}(t-1)}}$, calling $\widehat{\mu}_{i,a_i}(t)$ is the empirical mean of the observations for the ith component of the observation vector determined by the action component a_i, and $N_{i,a_i}(t)$ is the number of times the such a component has been played. Once we selected the best action according to our optimistic criterion, we play it and retrieve the observation vector $\mathbf{x}(t) = (x_1(t), \ldots, x_d(t))$. We use the observation vector to update the estimators and the related counters.

Regret Guarantees. F-UCB presents a worst-case upper bound as follows:

$$\mathbb{E}[R(\text{F-UCB}, T)] \leq \tilde{O}\left(\sigma \sum_{i \in [\![d]\!]} \sqrt{T k_i}\right).$$

5 Conclusions

We presented three MAB settings for dynamic pricing and advertising budget optimization. In Sect. 2, we proposed a model that allows us to model temporal dependencies in pricing through AR processes. In Sect. 3, we faced an advertising problem, and we focused on a new model to optimize MMMs. In Sect. 4, we proposed a model to optimize pricing and advertising coherently. For every scenario, we presented an algorithm to handle it, and we discussed its theoretical guarantees.

References

1. F. Bacchiocchi, G. Genalti, D. Maran, M. Mussi, M. Restelli, N. Gatti, A.M. Metelli, Autoregressive bandits, in *International Conference on Artificial Intelligence and Statistics (AISTATS)* (2024)
2. T. Lattimore, C, Szepesvári, *Bandit Algorithms* (Cambridge University Press, 2020)
3. M. Mussi, A.M. Metelli, M. Restelli, Dynamical linear bandits, in *International Conference on Machine Learning (ICML)* (2023)
4. M. Mussi, S. Drago, M. Restelli, A.M. Metelli, Factored-reward bandits with intermediate observations, in *International Conference on Machine Learning (ICML)* (2024)
5. M. Mussi, S. Drago, M. Restelli, A. M. Metelli, Factored-reward bandits with intermediate observations: Regret minimization and best arm identification. *Artif. Intell.* **347**, 104362 (2025)
6. M. Mussi, *Online Learning Methods for Pricing and Advertising*, Ph.D. thesis, Politecnico di Milano (2023)
7. M. Mussi, G. Genalti, F. Trovò, A. Nuara, N. Gatti, M. Restelli, Pricing the long tail by explainable product aggregation and monotonic bandits, in *ACM Conference on Knowledge Discovery and Data Mining (KDD)* (2022)
8. D. Court, D. Elzinga, S. Mulder, O. Vetvik, The consumer decision journey. *McKinsey Quarterly* (2009)
9. O. Chapelle, Modeling delayed feedback in display advertising, in *ACM Conference on Knowledge Discovery and Data Mining (KDD)* (2014)
10. Y. Abbasi-Yadkori, D. Pál, C. Szepesvári, Improved algorithms for linear stochastic bandits, in *Advances in Neural Information Processing Systems (NIPS)* (2011)

11. P. Auer, N. Cesa-Bianchi, P. Fischer, Finite-time analysis of the multiarmed bandit problem. *Machine Learning* (2002)
12. S. Bubeck, *Bandits games and clustering foundations*. Ph.D. thesis, Université des Sciences et Technologie de Lille (2010)

Advances on Multi-fidelity Learning

Riccardo Poiani

Abstract Sequential decision-making problems are a major area of research in AI due to their wide applicability. In these problems, an agent interacts with an environment over time to achieve a certain goal, with the key challenge that each decision will influence future options and outcomes. While techniques like bandit algorithms and reinforcement learning have shown strong performance in several domains, they often require a large number of interactions with the environment to achieve satisfactory performance. In many real-world settings, however, imprecise but cheaper data (e.g., interactions generated by using a low-fidelity model of the environment) can be exploited to make the training process more efficient. This has led to growing interest in multi-fidelity learning, which seeks to improve training efficiency by combining high- and low-fidelity data. This work presents theoretically grounded methods for exploiting multi-fidelity data in general learning scenarios.

1 Introduction

In the last years, *sequential decision-making problems* have received significant attention in AI, as they model a broad spectrum of real-world problems. In these problems, an agent interacts with an environment over time to achieve a specific goal, and the key peculiarity is that each decision the agent makes will influence future options and outcomes. In this context, a large variety of general techniques have been developed over the years to address various challenges. These methodologies include Multi-Armed Bandit (MAB) algorithms [1] and Reinforcement Learning (RL) [2]. Although these techniques have shown promising results (see, e.g., [3, 4]), they often require a large number of interactions with the environment to achieve a satisfactory performance level. For example, state-of-the-art RL algorithms can require millions of interactions to achieve meaningful results in standard benchmarks. In many real-world applications, however, imprecise but cheaper data (e.g., interactions generated

R. Poiani (✉)
Bocconi University, Milan, Italy
e-mail: riccardo.poiani@unibocconi.it

© The Author(s) 2026

C. Cappiello (ed.), *Special Topics in Information Technology*,
PoliMI SpringerBriefs, https://doi.org/10.1007/978-3-032-12359-6_4

by using a low-fidelity model of the environment) can be used to improve training efficiency. For instance, in robotic manipulation, where an agent controls a physical system to grasp various objects, querying a high-quality simulator is expensive. Yet, a simplified, less accurate model of the system can often be used alongside high-fidelity data to make the training process more efficient.

In this context, *multi-fidelity* learning algorithms (i.e., methods that collect and exploit data of different quality) have recently gained attention, primarily in the field of Bayesian Optimization [5], as a promising option for balancing performance and learning efficiency. In this document, we explore multi-fidelity learning from *several novel perspectives*. Our primary goal is to enhance learning efficiency in sequential decision-making problems by understanding how to leverage cheaper, yet less informative data, which commonly appear in various scenarios.

1.1   *Outline and Contributions*

First, in Sect. 2, we study a multi-fidelity variant of the *Best-Arm Identification* (BAI) problem [1]. In standard BAI problems, the agent has access to a set of arms, each associated with a reward signal, and the goal lies in identifying the optimal arm (i.e., the one with the largest mean) while minimizing the number of interactions with the environment. In the multi-fidelity variant, instead, the agent has access to cheaper approximations for each arm that can be exploited to reduce the identification cost, i.e., sampling from these approximators introduces errors but it costs less. This model finds applications e.g., in simulation-based studies in physics. We develop the *theoretical foundations* of the problem [6], and propose a *provably optimal* algorithm to solve it [7]. Secondly, in Sect. 3, we study how to improve *Monte Carlo* (MC) [2] estimation techniques for sequential decision-making problems. MC algorithms are at the core of several successful RL methods. We study how to exploit a hidden, intrinsic multi-fidelity structure within MC Reinforcement Learning algorithms, that is the ability of an agent to truncate a MC trajectory to obtain a less informative, but cheaper, interaction with the environment. Specifically, we formalize this novel problem and propose and analyze an algorithm that leads to theoretical improvements over standard MC techniques [8].[1]

2   Multi-fidelity Best-Arm Identification

In the classical fixed-confidence BAI problem [9], at each round $t \in \mathbb{N}$, the agent selects one arm A_t among $K \in \mathbb{N}$ possibilities, and observes a sample X_t drawn from the reward distribution corresponding to that arm. The goal of the learning system is to identify with probability at least $1 - \delta$ the arm with the largest mean

---

[1] The formal proofs of all the results we present are deferred to the articles cited above.

using as few samples as possible.[2] In several practical cases, however, querying an arm to obtain a sample from the corresponding distribution might be expensive. For instance, in the context of physics simulation studies, where pulling an arm corresponds to the evaluation of a complex model under some given arm parameters, intensive use of computing power is required to obtain the reward we are interested in. Nevertheless, simpler and, consequently, cheaper and biased, models might be available to the agent. For this reason, we studied a multi-fidelity variant of this BAI problem, where the agent during each round chooses both an arm A_t and a fidelity M_t with the following trade-off: a higher fidelity gives a more precise observation, but has a higher cost. The goal is then finding, with high probability, the arm with the largest mean at the highest fidelity, while minimizing the total cost, i.e., the *cost complexity*. After formalizing the problem (Sect. 2.1), we present lower bounds on the cost complexity (Sect. 2.2) and then we present our algorithmic solutions (Sect. 2.3).

2.1 Formal Setting

A multi-fidelity bandit model ν with K arms and M fidelities is described by $K \times M$ probability distributions $\nu = (\nu_{a,m})_{a \in [K], m \in [M]}$.[3] We denote by $\mu_{a,m}$ the mean of the distribution $\nu_{a,m}$. More precisely, for each arm-fidelity pair $(a, m) \in [K] \times [M]$, $\mu_{a,m}$ is the mean value of an observation of arm a using fidelity m. Let $\mu = (\mu_{a,m})_{a \in [K], m \in [M]}$. Each fidelity $m \in [M]$ is related to a certain concept of cost and precision. Specifically, each observation gathered at a fidelity $m \in [M]$ is associated to a known cost $\lambda_m > 0$; we assume, without loss of generality, that $\lambda_1 < \lambda_2 < \cdots < \lambda_M$. Furthermore, to convey a notion of precision, we assume that there are some known values $\xi_1 > \xi_2 > \cdots > \xi_M = 0$ such that, for all arms $a \in [K]$, the vector $\mu_a := (\mu_{a,m})_{m \in [M]}$ satisfies $|\mu_{a,m} - \mu_{a,M}| \leq \xi_m, \forall m \in [M]$. We write $\mu_a \in \text{MF}$ to indicate that arm a satisfies these multi-fidelity constraints. During each interaction round $t \in \mathbb{N}$, the agent chooses both an arm A_t and a fidelity M_t, it pays a cost λ_{M_t} and it observes a sample $X_t \sim \nu_{A_t, M_t}$. The goal of the agent lies in reccomending which arm a has the largest mean at the highest fidelity M while paying the smallest possible total sampling cost. We denote the optimal arm by $a_\star(\nu) := \text{argmax}_{a \in [K]} \mu_{a,M}$ (often referred to as $\star$), and by $\hat{a}_{\tau_\delta}$ the final recommendation of the agent at the stopping time τ_δ. The aim of a MF-BAI algorithm is to guarantee that $\mathbb{P}_\nu \left(\hat{a}_{\tau_\delta} \neq a_\star(\nu) \right) \leq \delta$ holds for all the MF-BAI bandits ν. Among this class of δ-correct algorithms, we look for the ones that minimize the expected identification cost, i.e., the *cost complexity*, defined as $\mathbb{E}_\nu[c_{\tau_\delta}] := \sum_{a \in [K]} \sum_{m \in [M]} \lambda_m \mathbb{E}_\nu[N_{a,m}(\tau_\delta)]$, where $N_{a,m}(t)$ denotes the number of pulls of arm a at fidelity m up to time t.

---

[2] For completeness, we mention that the BAI problem has been studied in several variants, see, e.g., [10, 11] and references therein.

[3] We assume that each distribution belongs to a canonical exponential family.

2.2 *Lower Bound*

We first state a lower bound on the cost-complexity. The result specifies a minimum cost that any δ-correct algorithm must incur to identify the optimal arm.

Theorem 1 *Let $\delta \in (0, 1)$. For any δ-correct strategy it holds that:*

$$\mathbb{E}_{\mu}[c_{\tau_\delta}] \geq C^*(\mu) \log \left(\tfrac{1}{2.4\,\delta}\right), \tag{1}$$

where $C^*(\mu)^{-1} := \sup_{\omega \in \Delta_{K \times M}} F(\omega, \mu) = \sup_{\omega \in \Delta_{K \times M}} \min_{a \neq \star} f_{\star,a}(\omega, \mu),$[4] where, for all $i, j \in [K]$, $f_{i,j}(\mu, \omega)$ is given by:

$$\inf_{\substack{\theta_i \in \mathrm{MF},\ \theta_j \in \mathrm{MF} \\ \theta_{j,M} \geq \theta_{i,M}}} \sum_{a \in \{i,j\}} \sum_{m \in [M]} \omega_{a,m} \frac{d(\mu_{a,m}, \theta_{a,m})}{\lambda_m}.$$

where $d(p, q)$ denotes the KL divergence between distributions p and q.

In Theorem 1, the quantity $C^*(\mu)$ describes the cost complexity of a multi-fidelity BAI problem μ as a max-min game where the max-player chooses a vector $\omega \in \Delta_{K \times M}$, and then the min-player selects a bandit model θ in which the optimal arm is different, with the goal of minimizing the function $F(\omega, \mu)$. The optimal vector ω^* that attains the maximum of $F(\cdot, \mu)$ can be interpreted as the vector of cost-proportions that an (oracle) agent should use in order to identify $\star$ by paying the smallest total cost.

To provide further interpretation on the complexity of MF-bandits, we derive the following additional result.

Theorem 2 *Consider a multi-fidelity bandit with Gaussian distributions with unitary variance such that for all $m \in [M]$, $\mu_{\star,m} = \mu_{\star,M} - \xi_m$ and $\mu_{i,m} = \mu_{i,M} + \xi_m$ for $i \neq \star$. Then, it holds that:*

$$C^*(\mu) \geq \Omega \left(\sum_{\substack{i \neq \star}}^{K} \min_{\substack{m \in [M]: \\ \mu_\star - \mu_i > 2\xi_m}} \frac{\lambda_m}{(\mu_\star - \mu_i - 2\xi_m)^2} \right),$$

where $\Omega(\cdot)$ hides costant dependencies.

Each term $\lambda_m (\mu_\star - \mu_i - 2\xi_m)^{-2}$ can be interpreted as the cost that is necessary to identify that $i \neq \star$ is a sub-optimal arm using samples collected at fidelity m only. Thus, the minimum over the different fidelities expresses the fact that, to conclude that the i-th arm is sub-optimal, one might solely rely on samples that are coming from (unknown) "optimal" fidelity (i.e., the one that is more cost-effective w.r.t. the bias ξ_m that the fidelity introduces). We note that only a subset of fidelities is present in the minimization, i.e., the ones that guarantees that $\mu_\star - \mu_i > 2\xi_m$ holds. Indeed, if a fidelity introduces too much bias it cannot be used to conclude that $i \neq \star$.

---

[4] We denote by Δ_n the n-dimensional simplex.

2.3 Algorithms for Multi-fidelity Best-Arm Identification

Starting from Theorem 2 and its interpretation, we derive a simple δ-correct algorithm, called Iterative and Imprecise Successive Elimination (IISE). Specifically, IISE starts from the cheapest fidelity, and it attempts to perform arm elimination using samples collected only at fidelity m. Specifically, IISE mantains a set of active arms $\mathcal{S}$, and during each round it pulls every active arm and it eliminates all the arms i such that there exists j such that the following condition holds:

$$\hat{\mu}_j(t) - U(t, \delta, \xi_m) \geq \hat{\mu}_i(t) + U(t, \delta, \xi_m),$$

where $\hat{\mu}_j(t)$ denotes the empirical estimation of arm j at time t and $U(\cdot)$ is a confidence bonus that is used to take into account the uncertainty from the estimation and the bias the fidelity m introduces. IISE will switch from gathering samples at fidelity m to fidelity $m + 1$ according to some technical criteria which directly arises from the goal of identifying arms with the optimal fidelity that we identified in the discussion of Theorem 2. ISEE stops when $|\mathcal{S}| = 1$, and $\hat{a}_{\tau_\delta} \in \mathcal{S}$. Under certain technical assumptions, it can be proven that the sample complexity of IISE is upper bounded, with probability at least $1 - \delta$ by:

$$\widetilde{\mathcal{O}}\left(\sum_{\substack{i \neq \star \\ \mu_\star - \mu_i > 4\xi_m}} \min_{\substack{m \in [M]: \\ \mu_\star - \mu_i > 4\xi_m}} \frac{\lambda_m}{(\mu_\star - \mu_i - 4\xi_m)^2} \log\left(\frac{1}{\delta}\right) \right),$$

where $\widetilde{\mathcal{O}}(\cdot)$ hides constant and logarithmic dependencies. As one can see, the theoretical guarantees of IISE closely mimics the structure of the lower bound.

To close the theoretical gap (i.e., to exactly match the lower bound), we propose a second algorithm that is called Multi-Fidelity Sub-Gradient Ascent (MF-GRAD). This algorithm is strongly inspired by the lower bound of Theorem 1. Specifically, it relies on sub-gradient ascent in order to optimize an empirical version of the function $F(\cdot, \boldsymbol{\mu})$, where, at each step t, $\boldsymbol{\mu}$ is replaced with its empirical estimate. In simpler words, MF-GRAD exploits sub-gradient ascent to find a sampling rule that follows the optimal oracle allocation that we presented above. The algorithm stops using a GLR test [9] and it recommends the most appealing candidate from a statistical perspective. From a theoretical perspective, MF-GRAD enjoys the following property.

Theorem 3 *For any multi-fidelity bandit model $\boldsymbol{\mu}$, MF-GRAD is δ-correct and asymptotically optimal, i.e.,* $\limsup_{\delta \to 0} \frac{\mathbb{E}_{\mu}[c_{\tau_\delta}]}{\log(1/\delta)} \leq C^*(\boldsymbol{\mu})$.

Theorem 3 shows that MF-GRAD exactly matches the lower bound of Theorem 1.[5]

---

[5] The nature of Theorem 3 is asymptotic. In the future, it would be interesting to derive a finite-time analysis of MF-GRAD (as it is done, e.g., in [12]).

3 Truncating Trajectories in Monte Carlo RL

In Reinforcement Learning (RL) [2], an agent acts in an unknown environment to maximize/estimate the infinite expected discounted sum of an external reward signal, i.e., the expected return. Monte Carlo (MC) evaluation [2] is at the core of many successful RL algorithms. Whenever a simulator with reset possibility is available to the learning systems designer, a large family of approaches (e.g., [2]) that can be used to solve the RL problem relies on MC simulations for estimating performance/gradient estimates on the task being solved. In this scenario, since the goal is to estimate the expected infinite sum of rewards, the designer usually specifies a sufficiently large estimation horizon T, along with a transition budget $\Lambda = QT$, so that the agent interacts with the simulator, via MC simulation, collecting a batch of Q episodes of length T. In this sense, the agent spends its budget Λ *uniformly along the estimation horizon*. While these methods have demonstrated promising and impressive results across a wide range of applications, they usually come with high computational costs, which are largely influenced by the sample inefficiency of MC simulation methods. Thus, we explore how to mitigate this issue by leveraging the reset function commonly available in many RL simulators. In other words, we identify and seek to exploit a hidden, intrinsic multi-fidelity structure within Monte Carlo RL methods—namely, the ability of an agent to truncate an RL trajectory to obtain a less informative, but cheaper, estimate of the policy return. After providing some background notion (Sect. 3.1), we lay down the theoretical foundations of the problem (Sect. 3.2) and we present an algorithmic solution (Sect. 3.3).

3.1 Background

We now present some background that is necessary to properly formalize the problem of truncating trajectories. A Markov Decision Process (MDP) [2] is defined as a tuple $\mathcal{M} = (\mathcal{S}, \mathcal{A}, p, r, \gamma, \nu)$, where $\mathcal{S}$ and $\mathcal{A}$ are the set of states and actions respectively, $p : \mathcal{S} \times \mathcal{A} \rightarrow \Delta(\mathcal{S})^6$ is the transition probability matrix that encodes the probability over the next states $p(\cdot|s, a)$, when taking action a in state s, $r : \mathcal{S} \times \mathcal{A} \rightarrow [0, 1]$ is the reward function that describes the reward $r(s, a)$ received by the agent when it performs action a in state s, $\nu \in \Delta(\mathcal{S})$ is the initial state distribution, and $\gamma \in [0, 1]$ is the discount factor. The agent's behavior is modelled by a policy $\pi : \mathcal{S} \rightarrow \Delta(\mathcal{A})$ that, for each state s, provides a distribution over actions $\pi(\cdot|s)$. When acting within an MDP, the agent observes a state s and selects an action a based on its policy π, i.e., $a \sim \pi(\cdot|s)$. This action causes the system to transition to a new state $s' \sim p(\cdot|s, a)$, and the agent receives a reward $r(s, a)$. Since we are dealing with sequential decision making problem, we now introduce some notation for sequences of interaction steps with the environment. A trajectory of length h is a sequence of h interaction steps that the agent takes with the

---

^{6} Given a set $\mathcal{X}$, we denote with $\Delta(\mathcal{X})$ the set of probability distributions over $\mathcal{X}$.

environment, i.e., $\boldsymbol{\tau}_h := (s_0, a_0, s_1, \ldots, s_{h-1}, a_{h-1}, s_h)$, where $s_0 \sim \nu$, and for all $t \in [h]$, $a_t \sim \pi(\cdot|s_t)$ and $s_{t+1} \sim p(\cdot|s_t, a_t)$. Given a trajectory $\boldsymbol{\tau}_h$, we also denote by $G(\boldsymbol{\tau}_h) = \sum_{t=0}^{h-1} \gamma^t r(s_t, a_t)$ its cumulative discounted return. Finally, for any trajectory $\boldsymbol{\tau}_h$ of length h, we denote by $p_h(\boldsymbol{\tau}_h|\pi) := \nu(s_0) \sum_{t=0}^{h-1} \pi(a_t|s_t) p(s_{t+1}|s_t, a_t)$ the trajectory density function for trajectories of length h collected with policy π.

In the Monte Carlo *on-policy evaluation* problem, the focus lies in estimating the return of a policy π by collecting trajectories via MC simulation using the *same* policy π. The policy performance is evaluated according to the expected return up an estimation horizon $T \in \mathbb{N}_{>0}$, i.e., $\mathbb{E}[G(\boldsymbol{\tau}_T)]$, where the expectation is taken w.r.t. the stochasticity of the environment, the policy, and the initial state distribution. In the following, we will refer to this performance index as $J(\pi) := \mathbb{E}[G(\boldsymbol{\tau}_T)]$. The most common approach to estimate $J(\pi)$ using MC rollouts is to specify an interaction budget $\Lambda \in \mathbb{N}$ such that $\Lambda \mod T = 0$, and to collect Λ/T trajectories of length T with the environment via Monte Carlo simulations. Then, the agent outputs the following estimate of $J(\pi)$: $\hat{J}(\pi) = \frac{1}{\Lambda/T} \sum_{i=1}^{\Lambda/T} \sum_{t=0}^{T-1} \gamma^t r(s_t^{(i)}, a_t^{(i)})$. We will refer to this simple algorithm as a *uniform-in-the-horizon* Monte Carlo method. Clearly, this estimator is unbiased, that is $\mathbb{E}[\hat{J}(\pi)] = J(\pi)$.

3.2 Theoretical Foundations

We first lay down the theoretical foundations for studying how to truncate trajectories in MC methods. We introduce the concept of Data Collection Strategy (DCS) to model how the agent collects data within the environment.

Definition 1 A *Data Collection Strategy* (DCS) for a transition budget $\Lambda \in \mathbb{N}$ is defined as a T-dimensional vector $\boldsymbol{m} := (m_1, \ldots, m_T)$ such that $m_h \in \mathbb{N}$ for all $h \in \{1, \ldots, T\}$, and $\sum_{h=1}^{T} m_h h = \Lambda$.

Each m_h represents the number of trajectories of length h that the agent collects in the environment, while the constraint $\sum_{h=1}^{T} m_h h = \Lambda$ encodes the fact the agent is collecting Λ interaction steps within the environment. We note that there is a tight relationship between $\boldsymbol{m}$ and the total number of samples that the agent collects at step t. In particular, let $\boldsymbol{n} := (n_0, \ldots, n_{T-1})$ be the T-dimensional vector where each component n_t represents the number of samples collected at time t. Then, we have that $n_t = m_t$, if $t = T - 1$, and $n_t = n_{t+1} + m_{t+1}$ otherwise.

Given the DCS formalism, we consider the on-policy evaluation problem of estimating $J(\pi)$. First, fixed any DCS $\boldsymbol{m}$, we discuss how to levarage a dataset $\mathcal{D} := \{\{\boldsymbol{\tau}_h^{(i)}\}_{i=1}^{m_h}\}_{h=1}^{T}$ of trajectories of different lenghts to build an estimator $\hat{J}_{\boldsymbol{m}}(\pi)$ of $J(\pi)$. We propose and analyze the following estimator, which enjoys several interesting properties (which we present later):

$$\hat{J}_{\boldsymbol{m}}(\pi) := \sum_{h=1}^{T} \sum_{i=1}^{m_h} \sum_{t=0}^{h-1} \gamma^t \frac{r(s_t^{(i)}, a_t^{(i)})}{n_t}. \tag{2}$$

Equation (2) sums over all the possible trajectories' length up to T (i.e., the most external summation), and over the collected trajectories of a given length h (i.e., $\sum_{i=1}^{m_h}$), the observed truncated empirical return, in which each reward at each step t is divided by the number of samples n_t that the agent has collected using the DCS m. Dividing by n_t takes into account that more data have been collected for certain timesteps. We now highlight a couple of interesting features of the proposed estimator. First, we note that Eq. (2) properly generalizes the usual Monte Carlo on-policy estimator of $J(\pi)$. Indeed, whenever $m = \left(0, \ldots, 0, \frac{\Lambda}{T}\right)$ (i.e., the uniform-in-the-horizon DCS), Eq. (2) exactly reduces to the usual Monte Carlo estimator. Second, we analyze the expected value of the estimator. Specifically, it is possible to prove that for any fixed m such that $m_T \geq 1$[7] we have that Eq. (2) is an unbiased estimate of $J(\pi)$, i.e., $\mathbb{E}[\hat{J}_m(\pi)] = J(\pi)$.

3.3 An Algorithm for Truncating Trajectories

We now present a theoretically grounded algorithm for truncating trajectories. To investigate alternative budget allocation strategies, we provide a generalization of the Hoeffding confidence intervals for the estimator that we proposed in Eq. (2), and we frame our goal as finding the DCS that minimizes such intervals.[8]

Theorem 4 *Let m such that $m_T \geq 1$, and $\delta \in (0, 1)$. Then, with probability at least $1 - \delta$ it holds that:*

$$\left|\hat{J}_m(\pi) - J(\pi)\right| \leq \sqrt{\frac{1}{2} \log\left(\frac{2}{\delta}\right) \sum_{t=0}^{T-1} \frac{c_t}{n_t}}, \tag{3}$$

where $c_t = \frac{\gamma^t(\gamma^t + \gamma^{t+1} - 2\gamma^T)}{1-\gamma}$.

Since c_t is a decreasing function of t, it is direct to see that to minimize Eq. 3 it is provably convenient to allocate more data to the first interaction steps.[9] Given Theorem 4, our algorithm consists in using as DCS the one that minimizes Eq. (3). Specifically, in [8], we derive *in closed-form*, an approximately optimal DCS (which we denote by $\tilde{m}^*$) that obtains, up to a constant multiplicative factor of $\sqrt{2}$, the optimal value of the objective function of interests (i.e., Eq. (3)). Furthermore, to understand the theoretical improvements of $\tilde{m}^*$ against the usual-in-the-horizon algorithm, we resort to Probabilistic Approximately Correct (PAC) analysis. Specifically, given an accuracy level $\epsilon > 0$ and a maximum risk parameter $\delta \in (0, 1)$, we aim at answering

---

[7] This is a mild requirement that simply demands that at least 1 sample for each interaction step.

[8] We note that minimizing confidence intervals is one possible choiche. In [13] we investigate how to truncate trajectories to directly minimize the estimation error.

[9] This result should not be surprising. Indeed, due to the discount factor γ, initial timesteps are more relevant within the expression of $J(\pi)$.

the following question: which is the minimum amount of optimization budget Λ such that $|\hat{J}_m(\pi) - J(\pi)| \leq \epsilon$ holds with probability at least $1 - \delta$? For what concerns the uniform DCS, by directly applying Hoeffding inequality, one obtains that $\Lambda = \mathcal{O}\left(\frac{T \log(2/\delta)}{(1-\gamma)^2 \epsilon^2}\right)$ is sufficient to satisfy the aforementioned PAC requirement. For $\tilde{m}^*$, instead, it sufficies: $\Lambda = \mathcal{O}\left(\min\left\{\frac{T \log(2/\delta)}{(1-\gamma)^2}, \frac{\log(2/\delta)}{(1-\gamma)^3}\right\}\right)$. According to the value of γ and T, this can be significantly smaller compared to the uniform-in-the-horizon MC method. This, thus, establishes a significant theoretical improvement of our method over the usual approach that is used in the RL literature.

4   Conclusions

We presented two studies that combine multi-fidelity learning within sequential decision-making problems. In Sect. 2, we studied the multi-fidelity variant of the BAI problem. Our results close the theoretical problem for the asymptotic regime of $\delta \to 0$. In Sect. 3, we investigated how to truncate trajectories in Monte Carlo RL to obtain an estimator with stronger theoretical guarantees.

References

1. T. Lattimore, C. Szepesvári, *Bandit algorithms* (Cambridge University Press, 2020)
2. R.S. Sutton, A.G. Barto, *Reinforcement learning: An introduction* (MIT press, Cambridge, 1998)
3. Silver, D., Huang, A., Maddison, C. J., Guez, A., Sifre, L., Van Den Driessche, G., ... & Hassabis, D. (2016). Mastering the game of Go with deep neural networks and tree search. Nature
4. Poiani, R., Stirbu, C., Metelli, A. M., & Restelli, M. (2023). Optimizing Empty Container Repositioning and Fleet Deployment via Configurable Semi-POMDPs. IEEE Transactions on Intelligent Transportation Systems
5. R. Garnett, *Bayesian optimization* (Cambridge University Press, 2023)
6. Poiani, R., Metelli, A. M., & Restelli, M. (2022). Multi-fidelity best-arm identification. NeurIPS
7. Poiani, R., Degenne, R., Kaufmann, E., Metelli, A. M., & Restelli, M. (2024). Optimal multi-fidelity best-arm identification. NeurIPS
8. Poiani, R., Metelli, A. M., & Restelli, M. (2023). Truncating trajectories in Monte Carlo reinforcement learning. ICML
9. Garivier, A., & Kaufmann, E. (2016). Optimal best arm identification with fixed confidence. COLT
10. Poiani, R., Jourdan, M., Kaufmann, E., & Degenne, R. (2024). Best-arm identification in unimodal bandits. AISTATS
11. Poiani, R., Bernasconi, M., & Celli, A. (2025). Pure Exploration with Infinite Answers. arXiv preprint arXiv:2505.22473
12. Poiani, R., Bernasconi, M., & Celli, A. (2025). Non-Asymptotic Analysis of (Sticky) Track-and-Stop. arXiv preprint arXiv:2505.22475
13. Poiani, R., Nobili, N., Metelli, A. M., & Restelli, M. (2023). Truncating trajectories in Monte Carlo policy evaluation: An adaptive approach. NeurIPS

Electronics

Exploring the Future of Navigation: High TRL Piezoresistive MEMS Gyroscopes

Andrea Buffoli and Giacomo Langfelder

Abstract In the last two decades navigation applications, currently based on fiber optic and hemispherical resonator gyroscopes, have been leading the MEMS gyroscopes market and research, as they could greatly benefit from the inherent low area occupation, power consumption and cost. This manuscript discusses the efforts to enhance the performance of amplitude modulated mode-split piezoresistive gyroscopes to cope with the requirements of inertial navigation applications. The work starts from a temperature characterization of the sensors, as in the considered scenario environmental conditions usually play a large role. Then, near navigation-grade performance are demonstrated by coupling the gyroscope with a custom designed low-noise integrated circuit, implementing the drive loop, automatic gain control loop and an open-loop sense chain, while digitization, demodulation and data transfer are performed by an off-the-shelf lock-in amplifier. Afterwards, in order to allow a full market compliant validation of the sensors, a pre-industrial compact and stand-alone FPGA-based demonstrator has been developed to extend the technology readiness level, providing consistent results with higher fidelity. Further miniaturization is sought through a second generation of the integrated circuit that adds the demodulation and automatic quadrature compensation stages.

1 Introduction

In the last few decades the Micro-Electromechanical Systems (MEMS) industry and market have grown very rapidly both in terms of development and revenue. One of the leading sector of this industry is the MEMS inertial device branch. MEMS inertial sensors are, these days, omnipresent from low cost consumer market to more demanding fields as automotive, medical or industrial. Lately, a great effort is put both from industry and research in trying to push the limit beyond these applications

A. Buffoli (✉) · G. Langfelder
Dipartimento Di Elettronica, Informazione e Bioingegneria (DEIB), Politecnico Di Milano, Milano, Italy
e-mail: andrea.buffoli@polimi.it

C. Cappiello (ed.), *Special Topics in Information Technology*,
PoliMI SpringerBriefs, https://doi.org/10.1007/978-3-032-12359-6_5

for angular rate sensors and try to make MEMS gyroscopes a key player also in the tactical, navigation and strategic markets, which are nowadays dominated by ring laser gyroscopes (RLG), fiber optic gyroscopes (FOG), and hemispherical resonator gyroscopes (HRG). As a matter of fact, there are several indicators showing that the miniaturization and definitive SWaP-C (Size, Weight, Power and Cost) reduction of inertial systems in the navigation field will be possible only through the MEMS technology [1]. Gyroscopes are typically classified, according to their noise (ARW—i.e. minimum detectable signal) and bias instability (BI—i.e. stability of the sensor output over time) performance, in different categories (usually called grades): (i) consumer grade, (ii) automotive grade, (iii) industrial grade, (iv) tactical grade, (v) navigation grade, and (vi) strategic grade from lowest to highest performance. Table 1 shows the target requirements for the aforementioned applications, in terms of ARW and BI. It is worth to note that applications in the navigation and strategic domains also ask not only for high precision and stability over medium-short operating times, but also for longer time frames, where environmental conditions play a large role, thus asking for offset (ZRO) and sensitivity (SF) stability in temperature in the order of few tens of *ppm* (after calibration). As schematically shown in Fig. 1, currently only interferometric optical gyroscopes (FOG, RLG) and hemispherical resonator gyroscopes (HRG) show navigation and strategic grade performances. However, despite all the technological efforts to decrease their SWaP-C [2, 3] towards the market target they still come short in reaching the same area, power and cost efficiency of the MEMS technologies. MEMS gyroscopes performance have been consistently improving in the last two decades, now being fully compliant with consumer, automotive and part of tactical applications. Anyway, all the MEMS gyroscopes currently in the market all rely on capacitive read-out that comes with disadvantages such as: (i) area-sensitivity trade-off, (ii) large DC voltages needed and (iii) large dependence from capacitive parasitics and feedthroughs and their related drifts. As a consequence, classic capacitive read-out MEMS gyroscopes performance improvement is slowing down and near-navigation grade has not been reached in a compact and affordable package, yet. In the last ten years, the M&NEMS technology developed by CEA-Leti [4] have emerged, as a valid alternative to classic capacitive MEMS gyroscope, proposing a different read-out technique based on NEMS piezoresistive sensing elements connected to standard MEMS structures. M&NEMS yaw gyroscopes (out-of-plane sensitive devices) coupled to a dedicated discrete electronics based PCB have already proven to be the smallest footprint near-navigation grade sensor in the literature [5], with $ARW = 0.005°/\sqrt{h}$ and $BI = 0.030 - 0.015°/h$. Thus, this research work takes place in this challenging scenario and tries to prove that M&NEMS based gyroscopes can be considered among the main players for satisfying the industry requests. This is achieved by extending its technology readiness level [6] and passing from a laboratory based validation, exploiting discrete electronics and off-the-shelf instrumentation, to a compact and full-digital output pre-industrial demonstrator.

Table 1 Gyroscopes performance requirements in different application fields

Grade	Angle Random Walk (ARW)	Bias Instability (BI)
Consumer	$> 5 / \sqrt{h}$	$> 10°/h$
Automotive	$< 0.5°/\sqrt{h}$	$< 10°/h$
Industrial	$< 0.5°/\sqrt{h}$	$1 - 10°/h$
Tactical	$0.05 - 0.005°/\sqrt{h}$	$0.01 - 1°/h$
Navigation	$< 0.005°/\sqrt{h}$	$< 0.01°/h$
Strategic	$< 0.005°/\sqrt{h}$	$< 0.001°/h$

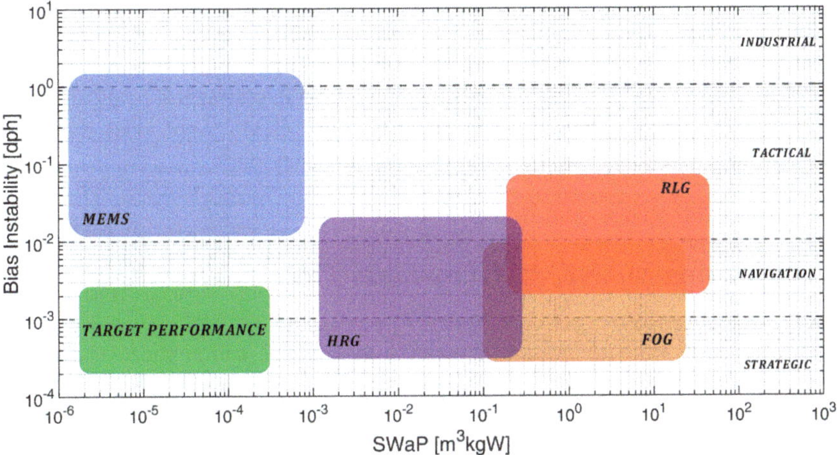

Fig. 1 Bias Instability and SWaP characteristics for the main gyroscope technologies, and in green the region towards which the market is trying to move

2 Thermal Characterization of M&NEMS Near Nav-Grade Gyroscopes

SF and ZRO thermal behaviour of MEMS gyroscopes is a critical topic, since they are sensors based on the coupling of different energy domains and because, depending on the target application, they may operate under severe thermal fluctuations that may range as wide as from $-45\,°C$ to $+125\,°C$. Therefore this section presents thermal characterization of yaw gyroscopes in M&NEMS technology, particularly referring to six samples showing near-navigation grade [5]. The temperature range explored during this measurement campaign has been limited by the climatic chamber capabilities to [5 °C; 85 °C] for the ZRO and by the rate table thermal range to [10 °C; 60 °C] for the sensitivity. No relative humidity (RH) control has been applied during these tests, with RH values ranging between 5% and 50%, typically showing an hysteresis behaviour between heating and cooling cycles. Results showed raw data ZRO drifts always below $580\,\mu dps/K$, with the best result being $75\,\mu dps/K$

and SF drifts between $180\,ppm/K$ and $850\,ppm/K$. Residuals after linear post-processing calibration were in the $\pm 5\,mdps$ and $\pm 1500\,ppm$ range for ZRO and SF, respectively. In terms of ZRO thermal drift M&NEMS gyroscopes show a $\approx$200-fold improvement with respect to uncalibrated commercial devices, and at the same time SF stability in temperature are in line with calibrated high-end devices [7]. Interestingly, a non-expected linear proportionality between SF value and its drift can be observed. Thus, a dedicated study has been conducted to address this trend. In the end, it has been demonstrated that this is due to the different role that the NEMS gauges play in setting the stiffness of the relative eigenmodes and the different Young modulus temperature coefficient for the NEMS and MEMS layers, resulting in a different temperature coefficient of the drive and sense modes. This in turn leads to a mismatch temperature coefficient inversely proportional to the mismatch value itself. Finally, as $SF \propto 1/\Delta f$, this confirms the observed $SF_{drift} \propto SF$ trend, which was also demonstrated by in-operation mismatch tracking experimental results [8]. This experimental campaign has thus confirmed that M&NEMS gyroscopes show very competitive performance also in terms of thermal behaviour.

3 Improving M&NEMS Gyroscopes TRL

In order to fully validate an inertial technology for high-end applications its TRL should be improved to confirm performance on a miniaturized integrated and digital-output system, which would also allow for vibration/shock tests and for real-time compensation techniques to fully validate its behaviour in operating environment. In this section two approaches for improving the technology TRL will be detailed:

- a mixed-approach solution employing a full analog low-noise integrated circuit (IC) developed for M&NEMS gyroscopes, coupled to a on-board A/D conversion stage and FPGA-based digital demodulation and signal processing;
- a fully integrated solution with an extended version of the same IC, integrating also the AQC and the demodulation stage, as well as a high-resolution ADC.

3.1 *Low-Noise IC for Near-Navigation Grade M&NEMS Gyroscopes*

In this context, a first version of a low-noise integrated circuit (IC) for M&NEMS gyroscopes has been designed. This IC implements: (i) the drive-loop needed to sustain the oscillation along the drive-axis, (ii) an automatic gain control loop (AGC) to regulate the drive motion amplitude x_D through a reference voltage $V_{ref,AGC}$ and (iii) an open-loop sense chain, exploiting the same analog front-end (AFE) used for the drive signal detection to minimize the demodulation phase error. Significant focus has been placed on the drive and sense AFE stage, as it must not introduce additional noise beyond the thermal noise of the piezoresistive gauges, arranged in a Wheatstone bridge configuration, and the thermomechanical noise of the sensor, respectively equal to $\left(6.3\,nV/\sqrt{Hz}\right)^2$ and $\left(8.5\,nV/\sqrt{Hz}\right)^2$ for typical gauges resistance and sense quality factor values. Three different AFE topologies has been carefully studied and designed and, in the end, a current-feedback intrumentation amplifier (CFIA) [9] has been chosen as the go-to option thanks to its better noise performance at equal power consumption, with respect to a classic voltage-feedback INA. Specifically, with the sizing of the implemented front-end, the input referred noise reaches a value of $\left(5.2\,nV/\sqrt{Hz}\right)^2$ with a total current consumption of 1.65 mA and a nominal gain of 21, sized to accomodate the maximum input signal coming from the sensor. An offset compensation loop has been also implemented at the CFIA output to compensate for any offset arising in the Wheatstone bridge due to mismatch in the nanogauges resistances, given by micromachining process non-uniformities, which can be as high as 5–7% of the nominal resistance. Figure 2 shows a schematic view of the designed $1.48 \times 1.47\,\mathrm{mm}^2$ IC, highlighting all the parts of the system which are integrated in the chip and the demodulation block and automatic quadrature compensation (AQC) loop, which are at this stage implemented through an off-the-shelf lock-in amplifier and discrete electronics, respectively. The IC and the MEMS dies have been assembled both in a stacked configuration, with bonding wires creating the needed connections between the two, and on different ceramic carriers,

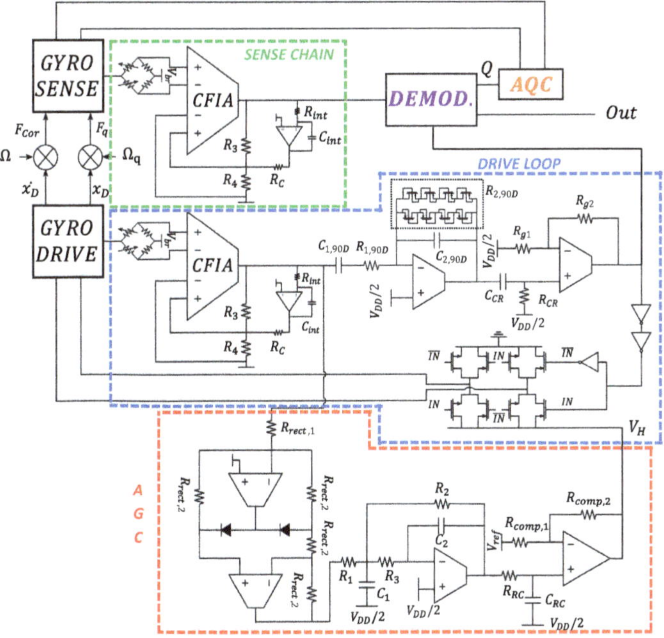

Fig. 2 IC block scheme

exploiting PCB interconnections between them. Thanks to the improved immunity to capacitive parasitics of piezoresistive-based gyroscopes, performance did not show any degradation between the two configurations. In detail, results [10] confirmed performance obtained with discrete electronics only in [5], showing a linearity error as low as $\pm0.2\%$ over a $\pm200\,dps$ full scale range (FSR), $ARW = 0.004 - 0.006\,°/\sqrt{h}$ and $BI = 0.02 - 0.03°/h$. All of this, while maintaining a current consumption as low as $6\,mA$ for the whole IC, in line with high-end power consumption limits.

3.2 FPGA-Based Full Digital Output Pre-industrial Demonstrator

After demonstrating that a custom low-noise IC allows to greatly reduce area occupation and power consumption, while not deteriorating performance, this section deals with the required steps to improve the technology TRL: implementing a standalone, full-digital output and compact industrial demonstrator. The first step in this sense has been the choice of the design methodology: an FPGA-based approach has been adopted, in parallel to the design of a second version of the IC (detailed later in Sect. 3.3), due its faster development, wide reconfigurability and easier re-design.

The conceived system, represented and pictured in Fig. 3, is composed by:

- a PCB hosting the M&NEMS gyroscope and IC coupling (in separate ceramic carriers), a temperature sensor, and carefully designed A/D sections in order to (i) digitize the sense and I/Q demodulation reference signals from the IC, while minimizing the introduced phase-lag through accurate PCB layout and (ii) bring back into the analog domain the quadrature compensation signal, connected to the quadrature compensation electrodes through specific buffers;

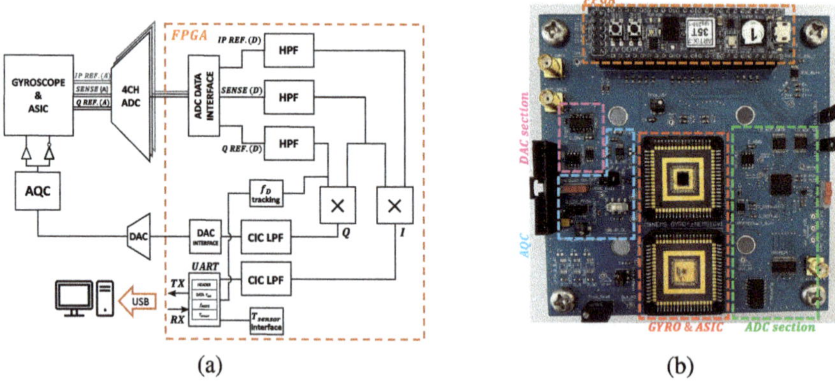

(a)   (b)

Fig. 3 High-level block schematic **a** and picture **b** of the conceived demonstrator

- an FPGA hosting the whole custom digital system, that includes (i) SPI interface to the system peripherals (ADC, DAC and T sensor), (ii) high-pass filters of the input signals to avoid residuals offset coming from the IC or the ADC section, (iii) digital signal multiplication to perform I/Q demodulation, (iv) CIC low-pass filters to attenuate spurious tones coming from the demodulation operation and reduce the output data rate, (v) a digital implementation of the AQC loop and (vi) UART communication through USB or RS422 protocol.

More details on the demonstrator design and characterization can be found in [11]. The setup, now consisting only in the previously detailed PCB, a $+5\,V$ supply (or battery) and a USB or RS422 cable, has been tested in laboratory and operational environment (also by a leading inertial navigation partner) in terms of sensitivity, linearity, temperature behaviour, turn-on/turn-on (T.O.T.O.) bias repeatability, and finally noise and stability through Allan standard deviation acquisition. The replacement of off-the-shelf instrumentation and/or components with custom designs have had no impact on performances, confirming once again sensitivity, linearity, temperature, noise and stability results detailed in Sects. 2 and 3.1. In particular, its worth to report that T.O.T.O. experiments have been conducted for the first time on M&NEMS gyroscopes, showing a turn-on/turn-on repeatability standard deviation of $1.12\,dph_{rms}$ over 50 system power-on cycles. Finally, Fig. 4 represents Allan standard deviations captured over 5 days of non-stop measurement (divided into fifteen 8-hours long acquisistions) in uncontrolled laboratory environment (with temperature variations within $\pm 2\,^{\circ}C$), showing $ARW = 0.006\,^{\circ}/\sqrt{h}$ and $BI = 0.016\,^{\circ}/h$, without any sign of drifts up to $\approx 3000\,s$ of observation interval ($\approx 10\times$ longer than previous discrete electronics implementation in [5]). To conclude, the proposed demonstrator shows performance metrics comparable with high-end products/prototypes present in the market/literature [11].

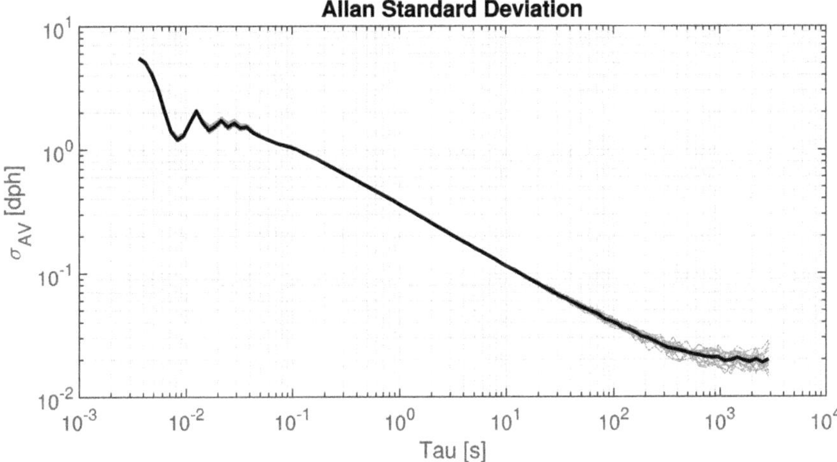

Fig. 4 Allan standard deviations calculated over 15 consecutive 8-h long acquisitions(grey dotted lines) and the average ADEV (black solid line)

3.3 Full System Integration

As anticipated in 3, an alternative path for improving the TRL of the technology, while fully preserving the advantage of MEMS technologies in terms of SWaP-C, is the development of the whole system in a single full-digital output ASIC. To that end, a second version of the IC has been designed by keeping the first version, detailed in 3.1, as the circuit core and adding the main missing blocks: (i) an AQC loop, with particular emphasis on the loop stability and the maximum compensable quadrature and (ii) a passive analog I/Q demodulation stage, featuring a delay chain to act on the demodulation phase error with a resolution of $0.1\,°$. The full analog $2.04 \times 2.17\,\mathrm{mm}^2$ ASIC schematic and picture can be appreciated in Fig. 5. The chip has been tested and validated in all its features, verifying their correct functionality, but unfortunately stability target performance were not reached due to a non-optimized stage in the output chain, introducing excessive $1/f$ noise. A re-design of the output chain has been assessed to reduce this excessive flicker noise contribution and the test chip is now in production. Conversely, the design of a high-resolution ADC to be coupled to this fixed release of the IC is still ongoing activity. Preliminary studies, supported by a thorough literature analysis, have highlighted the need for a $ENOB \geq 20\,bit$ precision and have delineated a second-order $\Sigma\Delta$ modulator as the preferred architecture for the analog-to-digital converter. No further details are provided at this stage, since design activity is still ongoing.

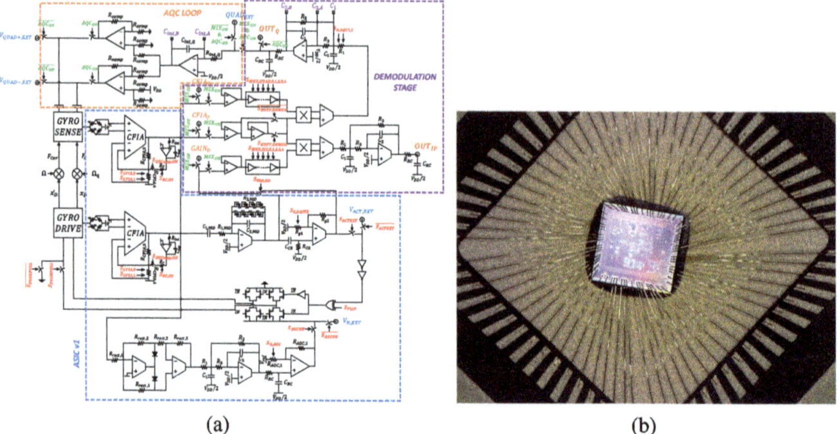

(a)   (b)

Fig. 5 Schematic (**a**) and picture **b** of the second version of the IC

4 Conclusions and Future Work

This chapter have presented the latest efforts to demonstrate that M&NEMS gyroscopes can play a relevant role in the inertial navigation field, bringing them from a laboratory-based setup to a pre-industrial demonstrator level. Near-navigation grade performance has been confirmed—also by an industrial partner—in terms of noise, stability, linearity, ZRO and SF thermal drifts and bias repeatability, while at the same time greatly reducing power dissipation and size, thanks to the development of a low-noise analog IC, coupled to a custom FPGA-based digital system. This step paves the way for a full validation of the M&NEMS technology, complying with the industry and market requests for a medium/high TRL prototype, which shows the sensors performance with high fidelity and repeatability grade. To conclude, it is worth to mention that pitch/roll gyroscopes (in-plane sensitive devices) in the M&NEMS technology have also demonstrated promising performance, among the best ever reported in literature for this topology of devices, with tactical-grade performance showing $ARW = 0.018°/\sqrt{h}$ and $BI < 0.2°/h$ [12]. Future work involves: (i) testing of the fixed release of the second version of the IC, (ii) design of the integrated high-resolution ADC to bring the gyroscope close to a final and industry compliant prototype, (iii) further work both in terms of characterization and design on pitch/roll gyroscopes, which still nowadays in the field are the main limitation towards a monolithic planar 3-axis tactical-grade MEMS gyroscope. Leveraging the results shown in this chapter and a decade long collaboration between CEA-Leti and Politecnico di Milano, the transition from laboratory to industry of the M&NEMS technology is now ongoing through a newly founded startup, iNGage.

Acknowledgements The authors would like to thank P. Robert, T. Verdot, P. Rey, M. Gadola, M. De Pace and P. Segala for their contributions and fruitful discussions.

References

1. G. Langfelder et al., J. Micromech. Microeng. **31**, 084002 (2021)
2. F. Dell'Olio et al., Miniaturization of interferometric optical gyroscopes: a review. IEEE Sens. J. (2023)
3. A.D. Meyer et al., Milli-HRG inertial navigation system, in *Proceedings of the 2012 IEEE/ION Position, Location and Navigation Symposium* (2012)
4. P. Robert, Piezo-resistive detection resonant device made using surface technologies. U.S. Patent No. 8,156,807, 17 Apr. 2012
5. M. Gadola et al., 1.3 mm^2 Nav-Grade NEMS-Based Gyroscope. J. Microelectromechan. Syst. (2021)
6. J.C. Mankins et al., Technology readiness levels, White Paper (1995)
7. A. Buffoli et al., Thermal characterization of scale-factor and zero-rate offset in near-navigation-grade nems-based gyroscopes. IEEE MEMS (2022)
8. A. Buffoli et al., Searching for the origin of zero-rate offset and scale-factor drift in nems-based nav-grade gyroscope. IEEE INERTIAL (2023)

9. R. Wu et al., Read-out integrated circuits, *Precision Instrumentation Amplifiers and Read-Out Integrated Circuits* (2013)
10. A. Buffoli et al., 0.02°/h, 0.004°/rth, 6.3-mA NEMS gyroscope with integrated circuit, in *IEEE Transactions on Instrumentation and Measurement* (2023)
11. A. Buffoli et al., Upgrading a gyroscope from a lab-based setup into a pre-industrial demo: challenges and lessons learned. IEEE INERTIAL (2024)
12. A. Buffoli et al., MEMS pitch gyroscope based on $(250\text{-nm})^2$ gauges achieving 0.12 °/h over 1000 dps full-scale. J. Microelectromech. Syst. (2024)

Updates and New Developments of the DAQ Firmware and Hardware for the EuXFEL's DSSC Camera

Andrea Costa

Abstract At the European X-ray Free Electron Laser (EuXFEL) in Hamburg, the DEPFET Sensor with Signal Compression (DSSC) project has built a megapixel X-ray camera that records images at 4.5 MHz, generating up to 134 Gbit/s. Its two-stage data-acquisition (DAQ) chain-16 Spartan-6 FPGA boards followed by four Kintex-7 boards—cannot satisfy future needs. Our work modernises this DAQ to future-proof the camera, simplify read-out, and boost performance. We began by analysing and refactoring the firmware and custom Linux build, eliminating faults, adding features, and improving robustness and ease of use. In parallel we evaluated replacement technologies, mindful that the current FPGAs are nearing end-of-life. Xilinx's UltraScale+ family emerged as the optimal platform, offering higher clock rates, larger logic and memory pools, and multi-gigabit transceivers with superior energy efficiency. A rigorous comparison of candidate UltraScale+ devices considered area, power, and timing. The selected chips provide ample resources for existing algorithms while opening headroom for future upgrades to the DSSC camera and other EuXFEL instruments. Deploying them will merge today's two DAQ stages into a simpler, faster, and more scalable architecture that sustains the 134 Gbit/s stream and beyond.

1 The DEPFET Sensor with Signal Compression (DSSC) Detector

The DEPFET Sensor with Signal Compression (DSSC) is an image detector designed specifically for soft X-ray detection [1, 2]. A novel strategy was employed to achieve high dynamic range and high gain for low signals, utilizing non-linear DEPFET

A. Costa (✉)
Politecnico di Milano – DEIB, Milano, Italy
e-mail: andrea1.costa@polimi.it

© The Author(s) 2026
C. Cappiello (ed.), *Special Topics in Information Technology*,
PoliMI SpringerBriefs, https://doi.org/10.1007/978-3-032-12359-6_6

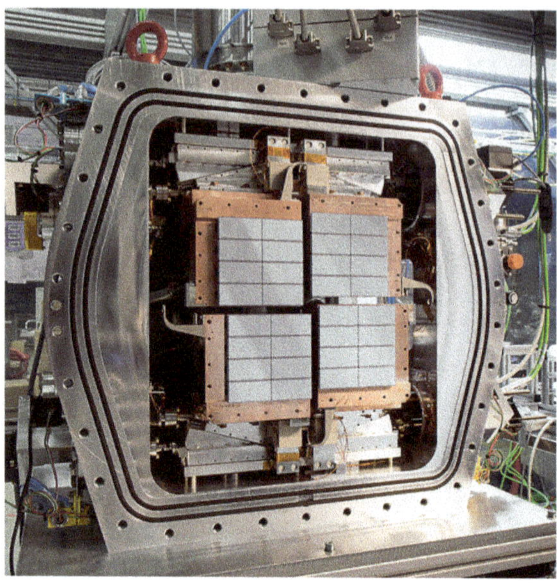

Fig. 1 DSSC camera and related mechanics and cooling systems

sensors. The fundamental characteristic of these is an extremely low noise, added to a response to the incoming signal which is inherently non-linear. The sensor can be read out by the front end built into the DSSC ASIC readout [3].

The ASIC handles readout, amplification, and analog-to-digital conversion. Additionally, the ASIC has a digital memory with a capacity of 800 frames. A matrix of 64×64 pixels is read out by a single ASIC. The fundamental component of a DSSC camera is the Ladder, handling 2 sensors (and related electronics) made up with 8 ASICs each, for a total 512×128 pixels. Adding together 4 ladders makes the so-called Quadrant. The DSSC detector is shown in Fig. 1.

2   The DSSC DAQ System

The Patch Panel Transceiver (PPT) [4] and the I/O Board (IOB) are two FPGA based sub-components of the DSSC DAQ system [5]. The IOB, shown in Fig. 2 is the first interface to the readout ASICs and is in the camera head inside vacuum. There is one IOB per module, i.e. 16 ASICs.

The PPT is the first element of the DAQ outside vacuum and serves one quadrant, i.e. 32 ASICs. The IOB reads out digital ASIC pixel data from the memory during the pause in between the trains and sends it to the PPT over fast data channels. The PPT PCB is visible in Fig. 3. It also handles low-level direct control of the sensor module electronics. For the crucial high-speed signals, special considerations in terms of

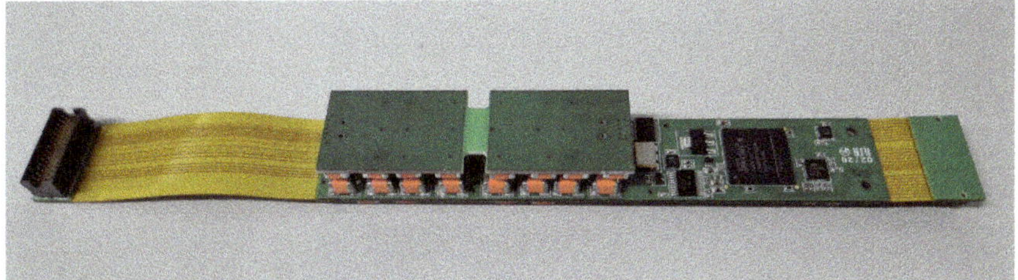

Fig. 2 IOB rev 1.1 PCB

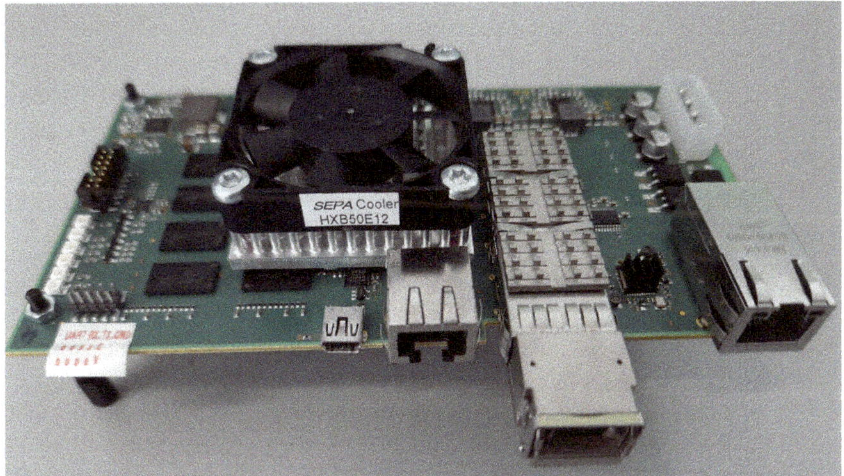

Fig. 3 PCB of PPT rev 2.1

signal integrity were developed for PCB layer stack-up and trace routing due to the dense implementation of the IOB. The PPT module is mounted on the outer backside of the vacuum vessel, outside the vacuum, and serves as an interface between the IOB and external subsystems. The PPT provides intelligent control for the DSSC instrument, handling one full Quadrant, i.e. 4 IOBs: it manages the data readout from the 4 IOBs concurrently, receiving it over twelve 3 Gbit/s links, buffering and reordering it into by leveraging on a DDR3 memory, and then sending UDP packets to the train-builder via four 10 Gbit/s links. The nominal bandwidth for payloads is approximately 4×9 Gbit/s.

As of today, we can assume that EuXFEL will continue operating as it does currently: the machine delivers 2,700 X-ray pulses per burst at a 10 Hz rate, resulting in 27,000 pulses per second being delivered to the samples under study and subsequently to the detectors. The DSSC, for its part, can store up to 800 images per burst, or 8,000 images per second, outperforming every other 1 MPixel detector at XFEL. In the near future XFEL is going to develop a new generation of detectors.

Table 1 Data rates of DSSC today (Now '20 s and the near future target for 2030)

Unit	Now '20 s (Gbps)	Target 2030+ (Gbps)
ASIC	0.31	4.54
Ladder	4.88	72.52
Quadrant	19.5	290.3
Camera	78.1	1160.16

The main idea is to reduce pixel size, keeping the same active area and therefore increasing the number of channels, probably targeting 4 MPixels $\times 4$ with respect to the current DSSC camera). With the assumption of the same continuous mode operation of today and the aim to use 10-bit ADCs, the data involved will change as reported in Table 1, considering the case in which all the 27,000 pulses/s are stored by the ASICs and transferred to the DAQ.

3 Quest for the Future DAQ System

The current IOB setup faces several challenges, including component shortages, operational limitations, and the need for more advanced processing capabilities. By addressing these issues, we aim to enhance the robustness, efficiency, and adaptability of the DSSC system. So, updating the IOB is essential. The new IOB should be equipped with DDR memory and a more spacious FPGA. This update will address current hardware limitations, enhance operational flexibility, and incorporate advanced data processing capabilities directly into the DAQ system.

In particular,

- By integrating DDR memory, the IOB will support real-time calibration, rebinning, ensuring optimal processing. A more spacious FPGA will provide the necessary logic capacity to handle standalone Ladder operations and implement complex algorithms directly on the DAQ.
- The updated IOB will be designed to ensure backward compatibility with the existing DSSC system. This means it can be seamlessly integrated with current setups, allowing for a smooth transition without disrupting ongoing operations or requiring extensive modifications to the existing infrastructure.
- These enhancements will make the DSSC system more robust, efficient, and adaptable to the evolving needs of scientific research, ensuring it can continue to deliver high-quality data while managing the challenges of component shortages, operational demands, and advanced processing requirements.

Once having defined the FPGA target device, which is the fundamental and most power-hungry IC of the whole IOB and estimated the firmware translation to the new technology, the following phase for the IOB redesign is the definition of the new Bill

Table 2 BoM comparison for the three possible new IOB solutions

	1-to-1 replacement	Additional features	Standalone IOB
FPGA	SU65P	SU100P/AU15P	AU15P
Renewed Hardware	Clk fanout, PMIC, LDO, XO	Like 1-to-1	Like 1-to-1
Additional Hardware	–	2 Gbit DDR3	2 Gbit DDR3, 1 Gbit DDR3, Flash, carrier board
Power Consumption	2.5 W	>3.2 W	7.5 W
Complexity	Low	Medium	Medium/High

Of Materials, with the intention of designing a completely back-compatible device there are constraints that must be respected, as size, total power consumption and total current consumption.

Considering the case in which the aim of the redesign of the IOB to produce spare modules is the only problem that needs to be addressed at present time, then the BoM would change accordingly to the previous section, featuring the following novelties:

- New clock fanout buffers
- New Crystal Oscillator
- Capacitor Bank replaced with an LDO regulator
- PMIC instead of single DC/DC converters.

This redesign allows for lower overall power consumption, ensuring a consistent power reduction leading to a secure utilization of the Peltier cooling for DSSC. The low overall power dissipation leaves space for integration of new firmware features, additions that are, in any case, constrained to the availability of FPGA logic for processing, and no external buffer memory to accumulate data throughout processing.

We have identified the target FPGA as the Artix UltraScale+ AU15P, with the possibility of downgrading to a smaller Spartan UltraScale+ SU100P for the only case of going for the additional features and not for the standalone IOB.

To address the needs for external memory support to allow accumulation of detector's ADC data before processing we considered the most available types of fast external memories. The images acquired by one quadrant are 512 kB each, and 800 images make up to 400 MB per train; as of today, the PPT features 1 GB of DDR3 memory to allow for buffering of two complete trains. When thinking of scaling down to a ladder, which is the sub-unit handled by the IOB, the memory needs are reduced to $1/4$, resulting in 256 MB, or 2 Gbit, which is a widely available memory size in single chip devices.

Table 2 reports a comparison between the various BoM configurations envisioned for the new IOB board.

4 Conclusion

Starting with focus on the DSSC camera, one of EuXFEL's 1 Megapixel detectors, the analysis revealed several hardware and firmware design limitations affecting its usability and performance. Effective solutions were implemented, notably the correction of timing misalignments among critical signals and data generated by the ASICs. The use of configurable FPGA resources enabled individual signal adjustments, overcoming the constraints of previous firmware implementations. A fast logic in the portion of firmware dedicated to the generation of signals to clear the DEPFET from charge during the bunch crossing extends the available delay range and significantly enhances the detector's imaging performance while addressing issues related to the DEPFET clear phase.

The inclusion of a DHCP server simplified the detector's integration within the EuXFEL environment. The most advanced scenario involves standalone operation with extensive feature development. In this context, the Artix UltraScale+ AU15P-2UBVA368 emerged as the optimal solution. It provides significant resource availability, including LUTs, FFs, and BRAMs, along with enhanced timing performance and higher clock speeds. Despite its higher static power consumption, its improved dynamic power efficiency and potential for advanced data processing make it a compelling option. Additionally, its scalability supports future expansions and technological advancements, making it the best candidate to replace the current Spartan-6 FPGA nearing its end of life.

The final option is a standalone-capable and 1-to-1 replacement BoM with external buffer memory and system memory for the MicroBlaze microcontroller. This configuration is built around the Artix UltraScale+ (AU15P) FPGA and gives hardware support for a completely new working mode, while retaining backward compatibility. Although this option has a higher demand, it unlocks extensive processing capabilities, making it suitable for future-proof, performance-intensive applications.

References

1. J. Sztuk-Dambietz, S. Hauf, A. Koch, M. Kuster, M. Turcato, in *Advances in X-ray Free-Electron Lasers II: Instrumentation*, ed. by T. Tschentscher, K. Tiedtke, International Society for Optics and Photonics, vol. 8778, (SPIE, 2013), p. 87780U. https://doi.org/10.1117/12.2020773. https://doi.org/10.1117/12.2020773
2. M. Porro, L. Andricek, L. Bombelli, G. De Vita, C. Fiorini, P. Fischer, K. Hansen, P. Lechner, G. Lutz, L. Strüder, G. Weidenspointner, Nuclear instruments and methods in physics research section a: accelerators. Spectrometers Detect. Assoc. Equip. **624**(2), 509 (2010)
3. P. Fischer, M. Bach, L. Bombelli, G. Vita, F. Erdinger, S. Facchinetti, C. Fiorini, K. Hansen, S. Herrmann, P. Kalavakuru, M. Manghisoni, M. Porro, C. Reckleben, pp. 336–341 (2010). https://doi.org/10.1109/NSSMIC.2010.5873776
4. A. Kugel, M. Kirchgessner, M. Porro, J. Soldat, T. Gerlach, in *2013 IEEE Nuclear Science Symposium and Medical Imaging Conference (2013 NSS/MIC)*, pp. 1–6 (2013). https://doi.org/10.1109/NSSMIC.2013.6829518

5. T. Gerlach, A. Kugel, A. Wurz, K. Hansen, H. Klär, D. Müntefering, P. Fischer, in *2011 IEEE Nuclear Science Symposium Conference Record*, pp. 156–162 (2011). https://doi.org/10.1109/NSSMIC.2011.6154470

Systems and Control

Meta-Learning for Data-Driven Control System Design: Theory and Applications

Riccardo Busetto⊙

Abstract This Brief shows how *similarity across dynamical systems* can accelerate data-driven controller and estimator design. Classical data-driven control (DDC) methods avoid explicit modeling but remain plant-specific and require costly re-tuning whenever operating conditions change. We propose two complementary strategies that exploit prior designs and perturbed training classes. First, **Meta-DDC** reuses controllers tuned on similar systems, and its extension **Meta-AutoDDC** automates the selection of the reference model. Together they guarantee non-deteriorating performance and improved robustness when designing controllers for unseen but related plants [4, 7]. Second, **in-context learning** with transformer architectures produces contextual controllers and estimators, trained on perturbed simulations to generalize across entire classes of nonlinear systems without re-training [5]. Experiments on brushless motors and nonlinear process benchmarks confirm faster design, reduced data requirements, and improved robustness. We conclude with perspectives on scalable, similarity-aware control design.

1 Introduction

Control systems are central to modern engineering, regulating physical processes from motors and robots to vehicles and industrial plants. Traditionally, controller design relies on accurate models, either derived from first principles or identified from data [15]. Yet modeling nonlinear systems is difficult, and small mismatches between model and plant can degrade performance. Since the true goal is the controller itself, this motivates *data-driven control* (DDC), which bypasses explicit modeling.

Seminal DDC methods include Iterative Feedback Tuning (IFT) [13], Virtual Reference Feedback Tuning (VRFT) [9], and Correlation-based Tuning (CbT) [14]. These directly tune controllers from experimental data, accounting for unmodeled

R. Busetto (✉)
IDSIA Dalle Molle Institute for Artificial Intelligence USI-SUPSI,Lugano-Viganello, Switzerland
e-mail: riccardo.busetto@supsi.ch

© The Author(s) 2026
C. Cappiello (ed.), *Special Topics in Information Technology*,
PoliMI SpringerBriefs, https://doi.org/10.1007/978-3-032-12359-6_7

dynamics. Later extensions introduced iterative optimization, notably Bayesian Optimization (BO) [2] and Set-Membership Global Optimization (SMGO) [17]. Applications include mechatronic systems such as BLDC drives [8]. Building on this, earlier work on the meta-extension of SMGO-Δ [6] showed how priors from related problems accelerate optimization. The present Brief extends this rationale beyond optimization, focusing on direct controller design and contextual learning.

In practice, many systems belong to a *class of related plants* sharing structural properties: BLDC motors of the same family, manipulators with varying payloads, or process units under different conditions. This motivates the central question of this Brief:

> *How can we exploit similarities across systems to accelerate the design of controllers and estimators?*

Recent machine learning suggests two complementary answers. *Meta-learning* [10, 18] extracts transferable knowledge from past tasks, enabling faster adaptation with limited data. In control, meta-learning has only recently been explored [12, 16, 19], and our contributions [4, 7] extend this rationale to direct DDC design via **Meta-DDC** and **Meta-AutoDDC**, which reuse previously tuned controllers and automate reference model selection.

A second, more radical approach is *In-Context Learning* (ICL), popularized by large language models [3] and recently adapted to dynamical systems [5, 11]. Here, a single model–typically a Transformer–infers the task directly from input/output trajectories, enabling contextual controllers and estimators that generalize across nonlinear plants without explicit re-optimization.

This Brief introduces the above rationale for data-driven control in two steps:

1. **Meta-DDC and Meta-AutoDDC** [4, 7]: meta-design strategies that combine prior controllers and automatically tune reference models, reducing experimental effort.
2. **In-context learning for control and estimation** [5]: contextual controllers and estimators based on Transformer architectures, applicable to entire classes of nonlinear systems without re-training.

Section 2 presents Meta-DDC and Meta-AutoDDC. Section 3 discusses in-context learning for control and estimation. Conclusions and open problems are outlined in Sect. 4.

2 Meta-Learning for Data-Driven Control

Classical direct data-driven control methods, such as Virtual Reference Feedback Tuning (VRFT) [9], can design controllers from a single batch of data. However, their performance depends strongly on user choices (e.g., the reference model), and they must be re-applied whenever the plant changes.

Our framework, **Meta-DDC** [7], addresses this limitation by reusing controllers previously tuned on *similar plants*. The idea is to construct a new controller as a convex combination of prior ones, with weights informed by similarity.

2.1 Meta-Controller Construction

Given N controllers $\{C_k\}$ designed for plants $\{G_k\}$, the meta-controller is

$$C(\alpha) = \sum_{k=1}^{N} [\alpha]_k C_k, \qquad [\alpha]_k \geq 0, \quad \sum_{k=1}^{N} [\alpha]_k = 1, \tag{1}$$

with closed-loop cost

$$J(C, G) = \left\| F\left(M - \tfrac{CG}{1+CG}\right) \right\|_2, \tag{2}$$

where $M(q^{-1})$ is the reference model and F is a weighting filter.

2.2 Theoretical Guarantees

Three properties (proved in [7]) formalize the benefits:

Proposition 1 (Non-deteriorating performance) *If $G = G_k$ for some k, then*

$$\min_{\alpha} J(C(\alpha), G) \leq J(C_k, G),$$

i.e., the meta-controller matches the best prior design.

Proposition 2 (Bounded loss) *If $G = G_k + \Delta G_k$ with $\|\Delta G_k\|_2 \leq \varepsilon$, then*

$$J(C(\alpha), G) \leq \sum_{k=1}^{N} [\alpha]_k \left(\tilde{J}_k + \mathcal{S}_k\right), \qquad \mathcal{S}_k \leq \|F \, \Xi^2 C_k\|_2 \varepsilon,$$

where $\tilde{J}_k$ is the cost on G_k and Ξ a stable operator.

Proposition 3 (Meta-stability) *If each pair (C_k, G_k) satisfies $\|\Delta_k\|_\infty < 1$ with $\Delta_k = M - C_k G \, \Xi$ stable, then any convex combination $C(\alpha)$ also stabilizes G.*

Together, these results guarantee that meta-controllers cannot underperform the dataset, degrade gracefully as plants differ, and preserve stability.

2.3 Data-Driven Reformulation

Since G is unknown, $J(C, G)$ is replaced with a VRFT proxy. From an auxiliary experiment with input $u^L(t)$ and output $y^L(t)$, the virtual reference and error are

$$r^L(t) = M^{-1}(q^{-1})y^L(t), \qquad e_v^L(t) = r^L(t) - y^L(t),$$

leading to the data-driven loss

$$J^d(\alpha) = \sum_{t=1}^{T} \left(u^L(t) - C(q^{-1}; \alpha)e_v^L(t)\right)^2. \tag{3}$$

Noise can be addressed by instrumental variables, and regularization terms bias α toward controllers with good past performance and high similarity. Thus the meta-controller is synthesized from experimental data alone.

2.4 Automatic Model Reference

A long-standing limitation of VRFT-based methods is the manual choice of the reference model $M(q^{-1})$, which specifies the desired closed-loop behavior. If M is chosen too aggressively, the designed controller may become unstable; if too conservative, achievable performance is unnecessarily limited. This design step often requires expert knowledge and trial-and-error.

In **Meta-AutoDDC** [4], the reference model is parameterized as $M(q^{-1}; \varphi)$, where $\varphi \in \Phi$ encodes admissible dynamic responses (e.g., desired settling time or damping ratio). The selection of φ is no longer manual, but posed as a *bi-level optimization*:

$$\min_{\varphi \in \Phi} J^{\text{auto}}(\varphi) \qquad \text{s.t. } \alpha^\star(\varphi) = \arg\min_{\alpha} J^{d,IV}(\alpha; \varphi),$$

where the inner problem designs the meta-controller for a candidate reference model and the outer problem evaluates both calibration performance and meta-information from past systems.

This automatic procedure aligns the achievable performance of the new plant with the prior experience encoded in the meta-dataset, avoiding unrealistic specifications. As a result, Meta-AutoDDC reduces user intervention, improves robustness, and better exploits the knowledge available from similar systems.

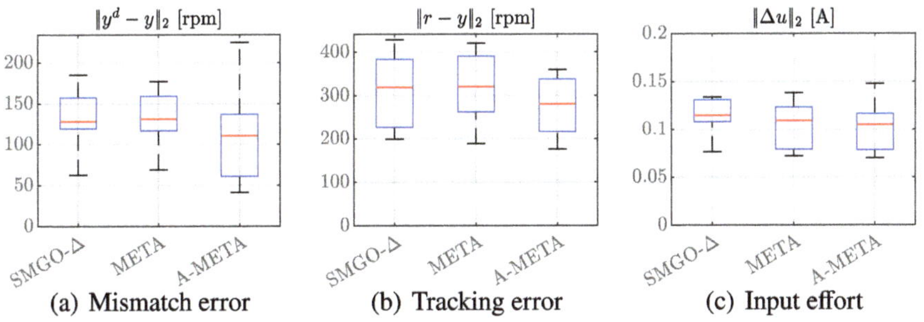

(a) Mismatch error   (b) Tracking error   (c) Input effort

Fig. 1 Comparison of non-flexible direct, data-driven techniques and the proposed meta-autoDDC approach: performance indicators across the test motors over 3 [s] long experiments

2.5 *Experimental Validation*

The proposed methods were tested on the tuning of PI speed controllers for BLDC motors within a field-oriented control scheme. The benchmark involved ten motor-load configurations for training and ten for testing.

Figure 1 compares SMGO-Δ, Meta-DDC, and Meta-AutoDDC across three performance indicators:

 (i) mismatching error $\|y^d - y\|_2$,
 (ii) tracking error $\|r - y\|_2$, and
(iii) input effort $\|\Delta u\|_2$.

Results confirm that:

- Meta-DDC achieves performance comparable to SMGO-Δ but requires only a single batch of data, rather than multiple iterations.
- Meta-AutoDDC further improves matching and tracking while reducing input effort, thanks to automatic reference model calibration.
- In contrast, VRFT (not shown) displayed higher variability and occasional instability, highlighting the benefits of similarity-aware meta-design.

3 In-Context Learning for Control and Estimation

Meta-learning accelerates adaptation across plants but still requires an explicit optimization step for each new system. A more radical alternative is *in-context learning* (ICL) [3], where a single model is trained across a class of systems and adapts on the fly from trajectories, without parameter updates or re-training. Recent work in system identification and estimation [5, 11] has shown its promise. Here we extend the rationale to both controller and estimator design.

3.1 Contextual Controllers

Consider a nonlinear system

$$x_{k+1} = f(x_k, u_k; \theta) + w_k, \quad y_k = g(x_k; \theta) + v_k,$$

where $\theta \in \Theta$ collects physical parameters (e.g., gains, time constants), and w_k, v_k are disturbances. At each step, the controller tracks a reference r_k using the context

$$\mathcal{I}_k = \{e_\kappa, u_{\kappa-1}\}_{\kappa=0}^k, \quad e_\kappa = r_\kappa - y_\kappa,$$

containing past tracking errors and inputs. A *contextual controller* C_ϕ maps this context into the next input,

$$u_k = C_\phi(\mathcal{I}_k),$$

where ϕ are model parameters (e.g., of a Transformer).

Generation of the meta-dataset. To build the training set, we define a class of systems

$$\mathcal{S} = \{(f, g; \theta) : \theta \in \Theta\},$$

obtained by perturbing the nominal parameters θ_0. Specifically, for each instance $i = 1, \ldots, N$, we draw

$$\theta^{(i)} = \theta_0 + \Delta\theta^{(i)}, \quad \Delta\theta^{(i)} \sim \mathcal{D},$$

where $\mathcal{D}$ encodes parameter uncertainties (e.g., uniform ranges, Gaussian perturbations). Each $\theta^{(i)}$ defines a new plant $G^{(i)}$ on which closed-loop trajectories $(u^{(i)}, y^{(i)})$ are collected. The meta-dataset is then

$$\mathcal{D}^{\mathrm{meta}} = \left\{(\mathcal{I}_k^{(i)}, u_k^{(i)}) \mid i = 1, \ldots, N, \ k = 0, \ldots, T - 1\right\},$$

where $\mathcal{I}_k^{(i)}$ are the context windows and $u_k^{(i)}$ the corresponding inputs. This synthetic procedure enables thousands of trajectories to be generated in simulation, covering the variability class of interest and ensuring reliable *sim-to-real transfer*.

Role of attention. Thanks to attention, the model weighs relevant portions of $\mathcal{I}_k$, using past input-output behavior as an implicit plant description This provides adaptation at inference time *without fine-tuning*.

The controller is trained against desired closed-loop trajectories $y^{d,(i)}$ from a reference model $M(q^{-1})$, by minimizing

$$J(\phi) = \frac{1}{N} \sum_{i=1}^{N} \sum_{k=0}^{T-1} \left\| y_k^{d,(i)} - y_k^{cl,(i)}(\phi) \right\|^2,$$

where $y^{cl,(i)}(\phi)$ denotes the closed-loop response of system i under C_ϕ. Once trained, C_ϕ can regulate unseen systems from $\mathcal{S}$ without re-tuning.

3.2 Contextual Estimators

State estimation is another fundamental task, typically addressed with Kalman filters that require models and careful tuning. We instead propose a Transformer-based *meta-filter* $\mathcal{F}_\phi$ trained directly from trajectories. Given context

$$\mathcal{I}_k = \{u_\kappa, y_\kappa\}_{\kappa=0}^k,$$

the meta-filter produces the state estimate

$$\hat{x}_{k|k} = \mathcal{F}_\phi(\mathcal{I}_k).$$

The training objective is

$$J(\phi) = \mathbb{E}\left[\sum_{k=0}^{T-1} \|x_k - \mathcal{F}_\phi(\mathcal{I}_k)\|^2\right],$$

computed from trajectories (u, y, x) of systems in the training class. At deployment, $\mathcal{F}_\phi$ generalizes to new systems in the same class without additional tuning.

3.3 Numerical Validation

We tested contextual controllers on the nonlinear evaporation process benchmark [1]. Figure 2 shows closed-loop responses for three representative test systems, comparing the contextual controller (ctx), an oracle MPC with known dynamics, and an identification-based controller (id). The contextual controller achieves performance nearly indistinguishable from the oracle while avoiding the identification step, demonstrating zero-shot regulation across unseen systems.

For the dual task of state estimation, we trained a Transformer-based *meta-filter*. Quantitative comparisons (Fig. 3) confirmed that the meta-filter consistently outperforms Extended Kalman Filters, even those using oracle models, by reducing estimation errors across 100 perturbed process instances.

ICL thus shifts the paradigm from "designing one controller per plant" to "training one model per class of plants". Figures 2 and 3 jointly illustrate how contextual models achieve both robust regulation and accurate estimation across perturbed systems, highlighting the potential of ICL for plug-and-play deployment in control and estimation.

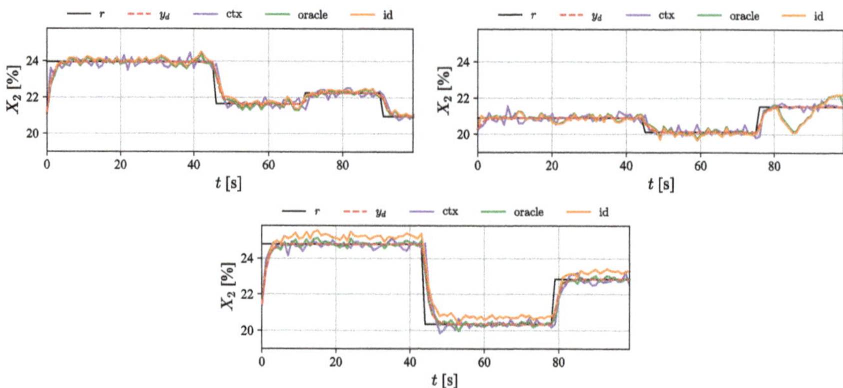

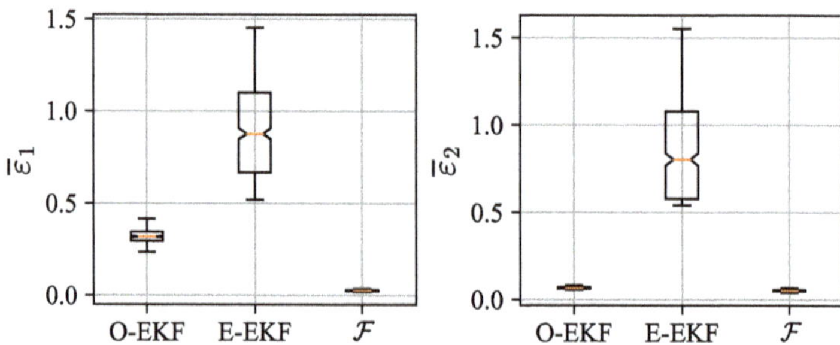

Fig. 2 Closed-loop responses attained by the contextual (ctx), oracle, and identification-based (id) controllers on three evaporation process instances

Fig. 3 Absolute estimation error across 100 perturbed evaporation processes: meta-filter versus oracle and extended EKFs

4 Conclusions and Future Directions

This Brief has shown how exploiting *similarity across systems* can accelerate data-driven control design. We presented meta-learning strategies for direct controller synthesis, including Meta-DDC and its automatic variant Meta-AutoDDC, which reuse prior designs and reduce the dependence on manual reference model selection. We also explored in-context learning with transformer architectures, yielding contextual controllers and estimators that generalize across entire classes of nonlinear systems without re-training. Experimental validations on brushless motors and nonlinear process benchmarks confirmed that these approaches enable faster design, reduce data requirements, and improve robustness compared to classical methods.

Future research should aim to extend meta-learning to a wider range of direct DDC techniques and validate them in industrial scenarios. Another promising direction is the development of hybrid strategies that combine meta-learning with model-based approaches, balancing performance, interpretability, and safety. Finally, advancing in-context learning toward truly plug-and-play controllers and estimators, with lighter training pipelines and mechanisms for lifelong adaptation, represents a key step toward scalable, similarity-aware control.

In summary, meta-learning and in-context learning provide complementary paths toward a paradigm where adaptation is an inherent capability of control design.

References

1. R. Amrit, J.B. Rawlings, L.T. Biegler, Optimizing process economics online using model predictive control. Comput. Chem. Eng. **58**, 334–343 (2013)
2. Berkenkamp, F., Schoellig, A.P., Krause, A.: Safe controller optimization for quadrotors with gaussian processes, in *2016 IEEE International Conference on Robotics and Automation (ICRA)* (IEEE, 2016), pp. 491–496
3. T.B. Brown, B. Mann, N. Ryder, M. Subbiah, J. Kaplan, P. Dhariwal, A. Neelakantan, P. Shyam, G. Sastry, A. Askell et al., Language models are few-shot learners. Adv. Neural Inf. Proc. Syst. **33**, 1877–1901 (2020)
4. Busetto, R., Breschi, V., Baracchi, F., Formentin, S.: Meta-learning of data-driven controllers with automatic model reference tuning: theory and experimental case study (2024). arXiv:2403.14500
5. R. Busetto, V. Breschi, M. Forgione, D. Piga, S. Formentin, In-context learning of state estimators. IFAC-PapersOnLine **58**(15), 145–150 (2024)
6. Busetto, R., Breschi, V., Formentin, S.: META-SMGO-Δ: similarity as a prior in black-box optimization, in *2023 62nd IEEE Conference on Decision and Control (CDC)* (IEEE, 2023), pp. 1294–1299
7. R. Busetto, V. Breschi, S. Formentin, Meta-learning for model-reference data-driven control. Automatica **172**, 112006 (2025)
8. R. Busetto, A. Lucchini, S. Formentin, S.M. Savaresi, Data-driven optimal tuning of BLDC motors with safety constraints: a set membership approach. IEEE/ASME Trans. Mechatron. (2023)
9. M.C. Campi, A. Lecchini, S.M. Savaresi, Virtual reference feedback tuning (VRFT): a new direct approach to the design of feedback controllers, in *Proceedings of the 39th IEEE Conference on Decision and Control (Cat. No. 00CH37187)*, vol. 1 (IEEE, 2000), pp. 623–629
10. C. Finn, P. Abbeel, S. Levine, Model-agnostic meta-learning for fast adaptation of deep networks, in *Proceedings of the 34th International Conference on Machine Learning*, vol. 70, pp. 1126–1135 (2017)
11. M. Forgione, F. Pura, D. Piga, From system models to class models: An in-context learning paradigm. IEEE Control Syst. Lett. 1–1 (2023). https://doi.org/10.1109/LCSYS.2023.3335036
12. T. Guo, A.A. Al Makdah, V. Krishnan, F. Pasqualetti, Imitation and transfer learning for LQG control. IEEE Control Syst. Lett. (2023)
13. H. Hjalmarsson, M. Gevers, S. Gunnarsson, O. Lequin, Iterative feedback tuning: theory and applications. IEEE Control syst. Mag. **18**(4), 26–41 (1998)
14. A. Karimi, L. Mišković, D. Bonvin, Iterative correlation-based controller tuning. Int. J. Adapt. Control. Signal Process. **18**(8), 645–664 (2004)
15. L. Ljung, System identification, in *Signal Analysis and Prediction* (Springer, 1998), pp. 163–173

16. S.M. Richards, N. Azizan, J.J. Slotine, M. Pavone, Control-oriented meta-learning. Int. J. Robot. Res. 02783649231165085 (2022)
17. L. Sabug Jr., F. Ruiz, L. Fagiano, SMGO-Δ: balancing caution and reward in global optimization with black-box constraints. Inf. Sci. **605**, 15–42 (2022)
18. J. Vanschoren, *Meta-Learning* (Springer International Publishing, Cham, 2019), pp. 35–61
19. L. Xin, L. Ye, G. Chiu, S. Sundaram, Identifying the dynamics of a system by leveraging data from similar systems, in *2022 American Control Conference (ACC)*, pp. 818–824 (2022)

Sparse Soft Decision Trees and Kernel Logistic Regression: Optimization Models and Algorithms

Antonio Consolo

Abstract Machine learning models have achieved remarkable results across domains such as healthcare, finance, and natural language processing. However, their adoption in sensitive applications often requires interpretable models, where sparsity can enhance both interpretability and generalization. We investigate and improve soft decision trees for classification and regression, which are interpretable models, and kernel logistic regression for binary classification. Contributions include new model variants, sparsification methods, theoretical properties, and decomposition-based training algorithms. For soft classification trees, we propose ℓ_0-based sparsification methods that are more effective in promoting both local and global sparsity compared to the previously proposed ℓ_1 and ℓ_∞ regularizations. For soft regression trees, we present a model variant where, for each input vector, the prediction is given by the linear regression associated with a single leaf node. We design a nonlinear optimization formulation amenable to decomposition and develop a convergent node-based algorithm that includes a heuristic for rerouting input vectors. Concerning kernel logistic regression, we develop a sparsity-inducing formulation for binary classification and design a convergent second-order sequential minimal optimization algorithm that achieves a good balance between sparsity and accuracy, while maintaining informative probabilistic outputs.

1 Introduction

During the past decades, the adoption and impact of Machine Learning (ML) models have grown considerably in many domains of society. However, many of the most powerful and effective ML models are inherently "black boxes" (e.g., deep neural architectures [15, 21]), which makes interpreting their outputs difficult. The widespread use of these black-box models, characterized by a huge number of param-

A. Consolo (✉)
Politecnico di Milano,Milan, Italy
e-mail: antonio.consolo@polimi.it

C. Cappiello (ed.), *Special Topics in Information Technology*,
PoliMI SpringerBriefs, https://doi.org/10.1007/978-3-032-12359-6_8

eters, primarily arises from their proven advantages in predictive accuracy compared to simpler and more interpretable methods.

Several ML models are applied in critical domains such as healthcare, credit access, employment, education, and criminal sentencing, where they help domain experts make decisions for which they carry full accountability. Therefore, it is crucial that those who use such models are able to interpret their results.

A model is said to be interpretable when it provides decision-makers with meaningful information about the patterns it captures and the resulting outputs [17].

Substantial efforts have been devoted to enhance the interpretability of ML models by leveraging the concept of sparsity [16], based on the epistemological Occam's razor principle, which suggests that the simplest model should be chosen among alternatives unless strong evidence indicates the need for a more complex one. Furthermore, simpler models are typically less prone to overfitting and therefore tend to exhibit lower generalization error, leading to higher accuracy on new data that were not part of the training set.

During the past three decades, there have been substantial improvements in hardware capabilities as well as in optimization algorithms and methodologies. These developments have led to several works attempting to leverage modern mathematical optimization to design novel methods for solving ML problems through Continuous Optimization and Mixed-Integer Linear Optimization (MILO) approaches.

A recent line of research has emerged that focuses on addressing ML problems through optimization techniques, highlighting the significant advantages that modern optimization methods can offer to the field. The application of mathematical optimization is crucial not only for training ML models with strong predictive performance but also for developing flexible solutions that consider interpretability and fairness. Several examples demonstrate how mathematical optimization can also help to interpret and visually represent model outputs (see, e.g., [10, 19]).

This work summarizes some contributions given in [7], where we investigate two supervised learning models, namely soft decision trees and kernel logistic regression. Decision trees are widely used ML models for both classification and regression tasks and are well-known for their high level of interpretability and good accuracy. Kernel logistic regression is a relatively less interpretable model used for classification task that extends the popular logistic regression by employing kernel functions. Given the importance of interpretability, the main focus is on enhancing decision trees. Special emphasis has been devoted to model sparsity, which allows not only to improve interpretability but also often to increase the testing accuracy.

In the following, Sect. 2 is devoted to soft decision trees. Specifically, Sect. 2.1 focuses on the classification task and presents an alternative sparsification method that achieves better performance than the original approach. Section 2.2 presents a more interpretable variant of the soft regression tree model, which is based on a nonlinear optimization formulation and is solved using a convergent node-based decomposition algorithm. Section 3 outlines a new nonlinear optimization formulation for training sparse kernel logistic regression. Finally, Sect. 4 provides conclusions and directions for future work.

2 Soft Decision Trees

In supervised learning, a training dataset $I = \{(\mathbf{x}_i, y_i)\}_{1 \leq i \leq N}$ is provided, consisting of N data points, where each $\mathbf{x}_i \in \mathbb{R}^p$ represents a p-dimensional feature input vector and y_i denotes the corresponding output value. In classification tasks, each input vector $\mathbf{x}_i$ is associated with a class label $y_i \in 1, \ldots, K$, where K denotes the total number of classes. In regression tasks, each input vector $\mathbf{x}_i$ is instead assigned a continuous response $y_i \in \mathbb{R}$.

A decision tree is a directed binary structure containing a set of branch nodes τ_B, including the root, and a set of leaf nodes τ_L. Each branch node has two outgoing arcs determined by a splitting rule. An input vector $\mathbf{x}$ is routed from the root through the tree by following the splitting rules defined at each branch node, until it reaches a leaf node where the output y, such as a continuous response or class label, is assigned. The splitting rule at each branch node can be either deterministic (hard) or soft (continuous), leading to deterministic or soft decision trees.

In soft trees, a sigmoid function is applied at each branch node to determine how a input vector is routed to the left or right branch. Specifically, for each input vector $\mathbf{x}_i$ and branch node $t \in \tau_B$, the probability of being routed to the left branch is defined by

$$p_{it} = F\left(\sum_{j=1}^{p} a_{jt} x_{ij} - a_{0t} \right),$$

where the coefficients $a_{jt} \in \mathbb{R}$ and the intercept $a_{0t} \in \mathbb{R}$ are decision variables, and $F(\cdot)$ denotes the sigmoid function $F(v) = \frac{1}{1+e^{-v}}$. Accordingly, the probability of taking the right branch is $1 - p_{it}$. Since the sigmoid function introduces a soft splitting rule at each node, all input vectors reach every leaf node with a nonzero probability. The probability that a input vector $\mathbf{x}_i$ with $i \in I$ ends up in leaf node $t \in \tau_L$ is expressed as

$$P_{it} = \prod_{t_l \in A_{L(t)}} p_{it_l} \prod_{t_r \in A_{R(t)}} (1 - p_{it_r})$$

where $A_{L(t)}$ indicates the set of ancestor nodes of leaf node t whose left branch is part of the path from the root to t, while $A_{R(t)}$ denotes the set of ancestor nodes whose right branch belongs to that path.

Figure 1 illustrates an example of a soft decision tree with depth $D = 2$.

2.1 Soft Classification Trees

In [1, 7], we investigate the nonlinear continuous optimization formulation introduced in [3, 4] to globally optimize sparse Soft Classification Trees (SCTs). In this section, we describe alternative sparsification methods that use concave approxima-

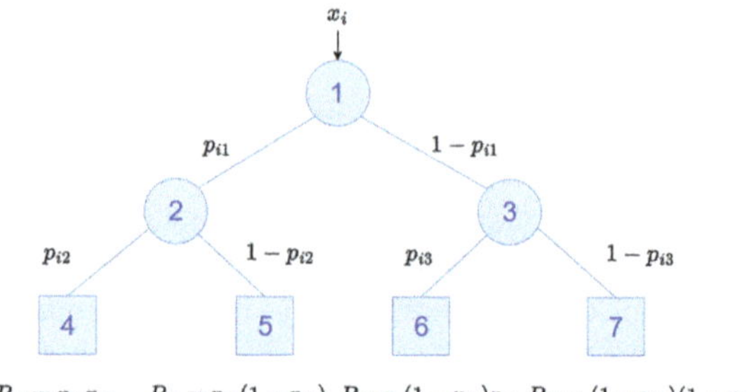

Fig. 1 A soft decision tree of depth D = 2

tions of the ℓ_0 "norm". For further details on sparsification, theoretical VC dimension bounds for multivariate SCTs, and a first node-based decomposition strategy, the reader is referred to [1, 7].

The SCTs described in [3, 4] are maximal binary trees with a fixed depth D, where $D \geq 1$. To address the classification task, it is necessary to define, for each leaf node $t \in \tau_L$ and class label $k \in 1, \ldots, K$, the binary variable c_{kt}, which equals 1 if all input vectors at node t are assigned to class k, and 0 otherwise. Moreover, the parameter $w_{y_i k} \geq 0$ represents the misclassification cost incurred when assigning $\mathbf{x}_i$ to class k. Minimizing the expected misclassification error is formulated as a mixed-integer nonlinear optimization problem with constraints requiring each leaf node to be assigned exactly one class and each class k to be associated with at least one leaf, while the integrality constraints on c_{kt} can be relaxed since the continuous relaxation yields an optimal integer solution (see [3]).

In classification trees, sparsity refers to the number of features used in the splitting rules at branch nodes. Two types of sparsity arise naturally: local sparsity, denoted by δ^L, which measures the average percentage of features not used per branch node, $\delta^L = \frac{1}{|\tau_B|} \sum_{t \in \tau_B} \frac{|\{a_{jt}=0, j=1,\ldots,p\}|}{p} \times 100$, and global sparsity, denoted by δ^G, which captures the percentage of features not used across the entire tree, $\delta^G = \frac{|\{\mathbf{a}_{j\cdot}=\mathbf{0}, j=1,\ldots,p\}|}{p} \times 100$. In [4], sparsity in soft classification trees is induced by adding to the objective function two regularization terms based on polyhedral norms of the parameter vector. Specifically, the ℓ_1 norm is used to promote local sparsity, while the ℓ_∞ norm enforces global sparsity.

To induce local and global sparsity in soft classification trees, we penalize the ℓ_0 "norm" of the parameter vector, which counts its nonzero components. Specifically, we add to the objective function one regularization term accounting for the total number of features used in the multivariate splits at branch nodes (local sparsity), and another term penalizing the number of variables involved across the entire tree (global sparsity). While ℓ_0 regularization provides a natural way to enforce local and global sparsity, it results in a nonlinear optimization problem that is more difficult to solve than formulations based on the ℓ_1 or ℓ_∞ norms, mainly due to the discontinuity of the ℓ_0 norm. Since the ℓ_0 penalties introduce non-smoothness, we use continuously differentiable concave approximations as in [6, 18, 22]. Nonetheless, in contrast to

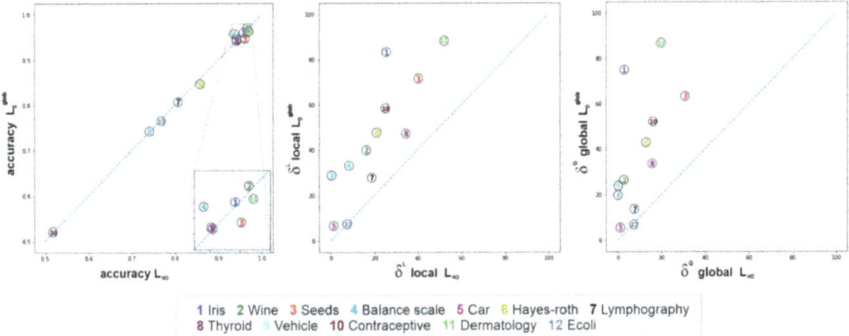

Fig. 2 Comparison of the global regularization proposals for 12 datasets in terms of accuracy on the left side, local sparsity in the middle and global sparsity on the right side. On the y-axis the L_0^{glob} model and on x-axis the L_∞ one

these works, training sparse SCTs does not lead to a globally concave problem. Therefore, similarly to [6], we replace the discontinuous step function $\mathbb{1}_{\mathbb{R}^+}(u)$ with the smooth concave exponential function $1 - e^{-\alpha u}$ defined for $u \geq 0$ and $\alpha > 0$.

We compare the ℓ_0-based sparsification method with the original ℓ_1 and ℓ_∞ approaches on 24 datasets varying in the number of features, data points, and classes. The reader is referred to [1, 7] for details on the experimental setting. Figure 2 from [1] shows the comparison between the ℓ_0-based approach (L_0^{glob}) and the ℓ_∞-based one (L_∞) on 12 multi-class datasets with $K \geq 3$ classes. The values for the ℓ_0 models are plotted on the y-axis and those for the ℓ_∞ models on the x-axis, with each dataset represented by a circle identified by a number. The results indicate that ℓ_0 regularization yields higher sparsity while maintaining comparable accuracy. In particular, in the comparison of global sparsity, the area above the bisectors in the middle and left plots shows that although L_0^{glob} and L_∞ achieve similar accuracy (as evidenced by the circles clustered around the bisector in the left plot), the former clearly outperforms in terms of both local sparsity δ^L and global sparsity δ^G. Overall, L_0^{glob} is almost always the best method with respect to both accuracy and sparsity.

2.2 Soft Regression Trees

To the best of our knowledge, the first formulation of soft regression trees was introduced by [20], where the authors referred to them as "fuzzy decision trees". More recently, in [5], the authors revisited the soft regression trees introduced in [20], with particular emphasis on promoting sparsity. In such soft regression trees, each input vector is associated with all leaf nodes, and the prediction is obtained by taking a weighted sum of the linear regressions corresponding to each leaf node, where each weight is given by the probability of the input vector falling into that leaf node. Since for any input vector $\mathbf{x}$ the prediction y is expressed as a weighted combination of the leaf node regressions, the final output of the tree is deterministic and hard to interpret. The trees in [5, 20] are equivalent to a mixture of experts, where each expert corresponds to the linear regression associated with a leaf node.

In [7, 8] we present a new model variant which offers several advantages in terms of both additional probabilistic information and flexibility in designing training algorithms. Specifically, our Soft multivariate Regression Trees (SRTs) define the prediction for any input vector as the linear regression assigned to a single leaf node, determined by routing the input from the root through the tree to the leaves. In this way, the prediction becomes more interpretable and the probability of reaching a specific leaf node t can be viewed as a measure of prediction confidence. Moreover, such SRTs exhibit the conditional computation property, meaning that each prediction relies only on a small subset of parameters associated with the nodes along the path from the root to the selected leaf node. This selective activation brings notable different benefits: it allows for faster inference, reduces parameter usage for each input, and serves as a regularizer improving the model's statistical properties.

By leveraging the conditional computation property together with an ad hoc objective function, we formulate a nonlinear optimization problem for SRT training that is well-suited to decomposition. We propose a general convergent decomposition scheme and a practical version that split the training problem into a sequence of subproblems, where at each iteration a selected subset of variables associated with nodes (the working set) is optimized while the others remain fixed. Decomposition methods are especially effective when subproblems exhibit favorable structures, as in our SRT training formulation, where minimizing over the leaf node variables while keeping the branch node variables fixed yields a convex linear least squares problem. At each iteration k, the decomposition scheme defines a working set containing indices of selected nodes, partitioned into a branch node set $W_B^k \subseteq \tau_B$ and a leaf node set $W_L^k \subseteq \tau_L$. For any node index t included in these sets, all corresponding variables are simultaneously optimized in the subproblem. Moreover, to promote balanced routing of input vectors along root-to-leaf paths, the decomposition scheme includes a rerouting heuristic that tries to balance the distribution of input vectors across the leaf nodes.

We also investigate the universal approximation property of our SRT, proving that any continuous function defined on a compact set can be approximated to arbitrary precision $\varepsilon > 0$ using an SRT of sufficient depth $D \geq 1$.

In [7, 8] we evaluate our SRTs on 15 benchmark datasets from a variety of applications. The results show that SRTs trained via the decomposition algorithm achieve better performance in terms of accuracy and/or computational time compared to two state-of-the-art methods: the nonlinear optimization framework for soft multivariate decision trees (ORRT) described in [5], and the deterministic regression trees (ORT-L) proposed in [2, 11] trained using a MILO-based local search method. Over all datasets, our SRT consistently achieves higher accuracy than ORRT, with gains exceeding 6% in 11 of the 15 datasets. Compared to ORT-L, SRT attains a higher testing R^2 (by at least 2% on average) and shows lower standard deviation, reflecting greater robustness to initialization. In terms of computational time, excluding datasets with small number of data points or features, SRT always requires less time than ORT-L. Finally, additional computational experiments indicate that adapting the decomposition algorithm to take into account group fairness constraints yields accurate SRTs that maintain similar performance across sensitive groups, without significantly affecting the computational load. The reader is referred to [7, 8] for a comprehensive discussion of the theoretical and experimental results related to SRTs.

3 Kernel Logistic Regression

Kernel logistic regression (KLR) is a popular supervised classification method used for both binary and multi-class classification problems, providing estimates of the conditional probability that each input vector belongs to a specific class. KLR generalizes logistic regression by leveraging kernel functions to represent complex nonlinear dependencies in the data (see e.g., [13]). In KLR, input data are mapped into a higher-dimensional feature space, where kernel functions define similarity metrics. In contrast to other kernel-based approaches such as Support Vector Machines (SVMs), KLR typically does not yield sparse solutions.

Over the past two decades, several approaches have been proposed to address sparsity in KLR. In [25], the authors introduce Important Vector Machines (IVMs), where sparsity in KLR is induced using a greedy sub-model selection strategy. This approach builds a proxy model by selecting a subset of data points in order to closely approximates the true hyperplane coefficient vector. To promote sparsity in ML models, regularization techniques such as ℓ_1, ℓ_2, and other variants are commonly applied. In [23], the authors implement an $\ell_{1/2}$-based method for KLR ($\ell_{1/2}$-KLR), leveraging the fast-converging half-thresholding algorithm introduced in [24], originally developed for a different family of loss functions.

The binary KLR model is trained by solving the following nonlinear optimization formulation:

$$\min_{\omega,b,\xi} \quad \frac{1}{2}\|\omega\|^2 + C \sum_{i \in I} g(\xi_i)$$

$$\text{s.t.} \quad \xi_i = -y_i(\omega^T \phi(\mathbf{x}_i) - b) \quad \forall i \in I.$$

where $\phi(\cdot)$ is the feature map which induces the kernel metric, C is the regularization parameter, and $g(\xi) = \log(1 + e^\xi)$ represents the negative log-likelihood (NLL) associated with the conditional probability:

$$P(y|\mathbf{x}) = \frac{1}{1 + e^{-y(\omega^T \phi(\mathbf{x}) - b)}}.$$

The similarity between the NLL loss in logistic regression and the hinge loss in SVM has been explored by several authors [14, 25]. However, unlike the hinge loss, which promotes sparsity due to its truncation property, the NLL does not exhibit this behavior.

In [7, 9], we extend the above formulation to promote sparsity in the model while preserving prediction accuracy. The objective is to modify the primal formulation so that the contribution of the NLL terms associated with easy-to-classify samples is reduced. The dual of this sparse formulation can be efficiently addressed using a decomposition method. Motivated by the decomposition method in [12] for SVM, we also design a Sequential Minimal Optimization (SMO)-type training algorithm that leverages second-order information and for which we establish global convergence. The key idea behind SMO-type algorithms is that at each iteration the working set consists of only two variables, which, in the dual KLR formulation, correspond to specific input vectors.

In [9], we present a comparison between our sparse KLR approach, denoted S-KLR, which is solved to optimality via the SMO algorithm, and other methods, including IVM, $\ell_{1/2}$-KLR, and SVM. The comparison is conducted on 12 benchmark datasets, focusing on test accuracy and sparsity. Experimental results indicate that S-KLR and SVM outperform IVM and $\ell_{1/2}$-KLR in terms of the trade-off between test accuracy and sparsity. As for the comparison between S-KLR and SVM, both achieve similar and significantly higher accuracy than IVM and $\ell_{1/2}$-KLR. S-KLR also provides substantial sparsity improvements over standard KLR. Although S-KLR is slightly less sparse than the inherently sparse SVM, this is compensated by the more informative probabilistic outputs of KLR.

4   Concluding Remarks

In this work, we presented improvements to soft decision trees for classification and regression, as well as kernel logistic regression for binary classification. The main contributions include the development of new model variants, theoretical results on the generalization capabilities of soft trees, sparsification strategies, and decomposition-based training algorithms to efficiently handle large datasets.

Given the critical role of interpretability, special attention was given to sparsity, which also helps improve test accuracy. In soft decision trees, sparsity was applied to the input features, naturally resulting in feature selection. In kernel logistic regression, sparsity was enforced by selecting a reduced set of data points, enabling faster inference and lower storage requirements.

Several lines for future work arise. For soft classification and regression trees, it would be interesting to explore alternative objective functions, deeper architectures with adaptive topologies, and improved decomposition algorithms with more sophisticated working set selection and initialization strategies. As to sparse kernel logistic regression, two natural extensions would be to address multiclass problems and induce sparsity with respect to the features.

References

1. E. Amaldi, A. Consolo, A. Manno, On multivariate randomized classification trees: l_0-based sparsity, VC dimension and decomposition methods. Comput. Oper. Res. **151**, 106058 (2023)
2. D. Bertsimas, J. Dunn, *Machine Learning Under a Modern Optimization Lens* (Dynamic Ideas LLC, Charlestown, MA, 2019)
3. R. Blanquero, E. Carrizosa, C. Molero-Río, D. Romero Morales, Optimal randomized classification trees. Comput. Oper. Res. **132**, 105281 (2021)
4. R. Blanquero, E. Carrizosa, C. Molero-Río, D. Romero Morales, Sparsity in optimal randomized classification trees. Eur. J. Oper. Res. **284**, 255–272 (2020)
5. R. Blanquero, E. Carrizosa, C. Molero-Río, D. Romero Morales, On sparse optimal regression trees. Eur. J. Oper. Res. **299**(3), 1045–1054 (2022)
6. P.S. Bradley, O.L. Mangasarian, Feature selection via concave minimization and support vector machines. ICML **98**, 82–90 (1998)
7. A. Consolo, Sparse soft decision trees and kernel logistic regression: optimization models and algorithms. Ph.D. thesis, Politecnico di Milano (2024)
8. A. Consolo, E. Amaldi, A. Manno, Soft regression trees: a model variant and a decomposition training algorithm (2025). arXiv:2501.05942
9. A. Consolo, A. Manno, E. Amaldi, *Binary Kernel Logistic Regression: A Sparsity-Inducing Formulation and a Convergent Decomposition Training Algorithm*. SSRN 5214848
10. S. Dash, O. Günlük, D. Wei, Boolean decision rules via column generation. Adv. Neural Inf. Process. Syst. **31** (2018)
11. J. Dunn, Optimal trees for prediction and prescription. Ph.D. thesis, Massachusetts Institute of Technology (2018)
12. R.-E. Fan, P.-H. Chen, C.-J. Lin, T. Joachims, Working set selection using second order information for training support vector machines. J. Mach. Learn. Res. **6**(12), 1889–1918 (2005)
13. T.S. Jaakkola, D. Haussler, Probabilistic kernel regression models, in *Proceedings of the 7th International Workshop on Artificial Intelligence and Statistics* (1999)
14. S.S. Keerthi, K.B. Duan, S.K. Shevade, A.N. Poo, A fast dual algorithm for kernel logistic regression. Mach. Learn. **61**(1), 151–165 (2005)
15. Y. LeCun, Y. Bengio, G. Hinton, Deep learning. Nature **521**, 436–444 (2015)
16. X. Li, Y. Wang, R. Ruiz, A survey on sparse learning models for feature selection. IEEE Trans. Cybern. **52**, 1642–1660 (2020)
17. W.J. Murdoch, C. Singh, K. Kumbier, R. Abbasi-Asl, B. Yu, Definitions, methods, and applications in interpretable machine learning. Proc. Natl. Acad. Sci. USA **116**, 22071–22080 (2019)
18. F. Rinaldi, M. Sciandrone, Feature selection combining linear support vector machines and concave optimization. Optim. Methods Softw. **25**(1), 117–128 (2010)
19. C. Rudin, Ş Ertekin, Learning customized and optimized lists of rules with mathematical programming. Math. Program. Comput. **10**, 659–702 (2018)
20. A. Suárez, J.F. Lutsko, Globally optimal fuzzy decision trees for classification and regression. IEEE Trans. Pattern Anal. Mach. Intell. **21**(12), 1297–1311 (1999)
21. A. Vaswani, N. Shazeer, N. Parmar, J. Uszkoreit, L. Jones, A.N. Gomez, Ł. Kaiser, I. Polosukhin, Attention is all you need. Adv. Neural Inf. Process. Syst. **30** (2017)
22. J. Weston, A. Elisseeff, B. Schölkopf, M. Tipping, Use of the zero norm with linear models and kernel methods. J. Mach. Learn. Res. **3**, 1439–1461 (2003)
23. C. Xu, Z. Peng, W. Jing, Sparse kernel logistic regression based on $L_{1/2}$ regularization. Sci. China Inf. Sci. **56**, 1–16 (2013)
24. Z. Xu, X. Chang, F. Xu, H. Zhang, $L_{1/2}$ regularization: a thresholding representation theory and a fast solver. IEEE Trans. Neural Netw. Learn. Syst. **23**(7), 1013–1027 (2012)
25. J. Zhu, T. Hastie, Kernel logistic regression and the import vector machine. J. Comput. Graph. Stat. **14**(1), 185–205 (2005)

Prosumer Decision-Making in a Carbon-Neutral Society

Araavind Sridhar

Abstract The increasing adoption of rooftop photovoltaic (PV) systems, electric vehicles (EVs), and electric heating positions the residential sector as a key provider of demand-side flexibility to support a sustainable energy transition. Demand response (DR) enables households to adjust electricity use to help balance the grid, but effective implementation relies on understanding how consumers decide to participate. This doctoral dissertation investigates residential consumers' decision-making regarding DR enrollment. The research identifies motivators across different socioeconomic groups, quantifies willingness to provide flexible loads, examines variations among household types, and models decision-making behavior mathematically. A detailed survey of Finnish households was conducted to assess motivations and preferences. The findings informed the development of an agent-based model that simulates how enrollment evolves over time. The study also proposes a pricing strategy for aggregators to attract residential flexibility cost-effectively. Results highlight that motivators such as financial savings, environmental awareness, and convenience significantly influence participation, and that willingness varies by demographic factors. These insights support DR service providers, policymakers, and researchers in designing more effective DR programs. By linking behavioral factors with system-level flexibility goals, this work offers practical guidance to maximize residential DR participation, ultimately contributing to a more resilient and decarbonized energy system.

1 Introduction

In the transition towards carbon neutrality, the residential sector is increasingly recognized as a significant source of energy flexibility. The proliferation of rooftop solar photovoltaic (PV) systems, electric vehicles (EVs), and smart electric heating systems through heat pumps (HPs) has transformed households from passive consumers

A. Sridhar (✉)
Politecnico di Milano, Milan, Italy
e-mail: araavind.sridhar@polimi.it

C. Cappiello (ed.), *Special Topics in Information Technology*,
PoliMI SpringerBriefs, https://doi.org/10.1007/978-3-032-12359-6_9

to active "prosumers". This shift offers new opportunities for balancing supply and demand in the power system through demand response (DR) programs, which rely on households adjusting consumption or injecting stored energy in response to market signals or grid needs.

However, achieving large-scale residential flexibility is not merely a technical challenge. It crucially depends on the willingness of households to participate, share control over their appliances, and trust third parties such as aggregators to manage their flexible resources. While technical solutions and economic incentives have been widely studied, there is still limited understanding of the behavioral and socioeconomic drivers that affect whether and how households engage with DR programs. This knowledge gap hampers the design of effective DR strategies and limits the potential to unlock residential flexibility at scale.

This thesis addresses this critical challenge by investigating how residential prosumers decide to enroll their flexible assets into DR programs. By combining survey research, statistical modeling, agent-based simulation, and pricing strategy design, this work contributes a comprehensive understanding of the motivational, behavioral, and economic aspects that underpin residential DR participation.

1.1 Research Objective and Questions

With the ongoing rise in rooftop PV installations and the growing share of electric vehicles, today's typical electricity consumer is increasingly evolving into an active prosumer. Unlocking the full potential of residential flexibility to support a carbon-neutral energy system depends on understanding how these prosumers make decisions. Based on this, the main research objective of the dissertation is:

Understanding prosumer decision-making in the future where the energy system will be carbon-neutral

In order to achieve the research objective, the following research questions are formulated:

- What motivates different socioeconomic groups to participate in DR programs?
- How can household willingness to enroll various loads in DR be quantified, and how does this willingness differ across consumer segments?
- How can prosumer decision-making for DR enrollment be represented through mathematical models, and how do adoption trends evolve over time?
- What pricing strategies should aggregators implement to effectively utilize residential flexibility while balancing profitability and consumer welfare?

By developing mathematical models of prosumer decision-making, this study sheds light on how enrollment patterns may change over time, providing deeper insights into future flexibility potential in the residential sector.

To answer the research questions, nine different publications are reported within this dissertation and an overview of these can be observed in Table 1.

Table 1 Overview of the dissertation publications

Pub.	Title	Overview
I	Assessing the economic and environmental benefits of residential demand response: A Finnish case study	Examines static and dynamic DR strategies in Finnish households, showing how consumer preferences affect cost savings and CO_2 reduction [8]
II	Residential consumer preferences to demand response: Analysis of different motivators to enroll in direct load control demand response	Identifies six main motivators for DR via survey; clusters consumers into subgroups based on motivators and sociodemographic factors [11]
III	Toward residential flexibility–Consumer willingness to enroll household loads in demand response	Quantifies willingness to enroll appliances, EVs, and HPs in DR; shows how socioeconomic factors and requested compensation influence participation [12]
IV	Nation-wide projection of motivators and consumer willingness for direct load control demand response in Finland	Extrapolates survey results to national demographics; estimates realistic residential flexibility for DR policy design [10]
V	The impact of an energy crisis on the residential consumers' consumption behavior based on a Finnish case study	Analyzes how the Russia-Ukraine conflict changed Finnish residential load shifting behavior [9]
VI	Residential consumer enrollment in demand response: An agent-based approach	Develops an Agent Based Model (ABM) simulating DR adoption based on financial/social factors; tested on synthetic neighborhoods with different DR contracts [14]
VII	Consumer enrollment in residential demand response: Implications across diverse societies	Uses the ABM tool to compare DR enrollment across three society types with different main drivers [13]
VIII	Residential demand response enrollment scenarios: A geospatial case study of Finland	Extends the ABM with Finnish geospatial data; shows regional DR enrollment variation over time [16]
IX	Aggregator decision analysis in residential demand response, considering consumer behaviors under uncertainty	Proposes a bi-level stochastic model for aggregator pricing in incentive DR; includes spot price risks and consumer uncertainty [15]

2   State of the Art

Supporting the sustainable transition of the energy system requires various strategies, among which Demand-Side Management (DSM) plays a key role in improving energy efficiency, reducing peak demand, and enhancing grid reliability [6]. DSM is broadly categorized into energy efficiency and DR. This dissertation focuses on DR, as it directly enables flexibility to balance intermittent renewable generation.

DR is defined as deliberate changes in electricity consumption in response to time-varying prices or incentives. It can be price-based–where consumers adjust usage in response to price signals–or incentive-based, where utilities or aggregators control loads directly (Direct Load Control, DLC) [17].

Across sectors, DR implementation varies. In the industrial and commercial sectors, several flagship pilot projects have been implemented in the recent times whereas limited participation of residential sector has been observed and large-scale participation in residential DLC DR remains challenging due to concerns around privacy, control, and trust [17].

To understand consumer preferences, choice experiments (CEs) have been widely used. Notable studies include Ruokamo et al. [7] in Finland, Broberg and Persson [2] in Sweden, and Yilmaz et al. [19] in Switzerland, highlighting that consumers favor financial and environmental benefits but often prefer DLC for heating over appliances.

ABMs have gained traction to simulate consumer DR adoption. Prior works modeled technology adoption for distributed energy resources [4] and DR in commercial settings [3], yet residential DR adoption simulation remains limited.

Finally, estimating available flexibility requires understanding consumer responses to incentives. Studies have analyzed baselines [5], utility functions [18], and price elasticity [1], but challenges remain in capturing real consumer behavior.

Together, this state of the art underlines the technical potential and behavioral barriers of DR, highlighting the need for refined models and better understanding of consumer motivators to unlock residential flexibility at scale.

3   Research Design

This dissertation explores residential DR adoption from technical, behavioral, and market perspectives, focusing on Finnish households and flexible loads such as EVs, heat pumps, and appliances.

The research is structured into three main themes:

- **Technical potential and benefits**: Using Mixed-Integer Linear-Programming (MILP) based optimization, the economic and environmental benefits of static and dynamic DR are quantified based on Finnish consumption data (Publication I).

- **Consumer preferences and willingness**: A large-scale survey was designed and distributed to capture residential motivators, willingness to enroll (WTE) in direct load control DR, and compensation preferences. Respondents were clustered by preferences and demographics; national-level projections were made via iterative proportional fitting (Publications II–V).
- **Consumer decision-making and market modeling**: An ABM incorporating financial and social influences on enrollment was developed and tested across different societal scenarios and geospatial datasets (Publications VI–VIII). Finally, a bi-level stochastic optimization approach models aggregator pricing strategies and consumer responses under uncertainty to evaluate DR feasibility and profitability (Publication IX).

Methods: This dissertation employed a mixed-methods approach to investigate residential DR participation. The consumer preferences and WTE in DR programs are estimated through consumer responses from a survey. Statistical techniques were used to identify consumer clusters with distinct socioeconomic and dwelling characteristics, which informed the segmentation of households for tailored DR program design. The ABM incorporates an MILP optimization to evaluate the consumer decision-making to enroll in DR based on economical and social factors. The ABM was further enhanced with sensitivity and Monte Carlo analyses to capture uncertainty and explore the impact of social influence and financial incentives on participation rates.

Data: The primary data source was a comprehensive survey targeting Finnish residential consumers ($\approx$ 30,000 Finnish households contacted, $\approx$ 1,468 completed responses). The survey gathered detailed information on household demographics, dwelling attributes, attitudes toward various DR motivators, and load-specific WTE for direct load control. This dataset enabled the estimation of preference structures and provided empirical inputs for the ABM simulation. In addition, literature-based estimates and publicly available energy market data supported the modeling of incentive pricing and aggregator cost scenarios.

Limitations: While the study provides valuable insights, several limitations should be noted. First, the survey data reflects the Finnish residential context; thus, generalizability to other countries may be constrained by differing social, cultural, and regulatory conditions. Second, the behavioral assumptions–such as price elasticity and the strength of social influence–are derived from literature and self-reported preferences, which may not fully capture actual consumer behavior in real-life settings. Third, the models have not yet been validated through implementation in full-scale pilot projects, and real-world complexities could lead to deviations from the simulated results. Finally, the current framework focuses primarily on spot-market price signals; the integration of additional market services, such as frequency regulation and ancillary services, remains a relevant direction for future research.

4 Findings And Contribution

This dissertation provides an integrated view of how residential households can contribute to DR in evolving electricity markets by focusing on consumer decision-making, flexibility potential, willingness to enroll, and modeling of adoption dynamics. The key findings are structured around five main research questions addressed through six publications.

First, the dissertation quantified the theoretical maximum savings potential achievable through residential DR under various scheduling strategies and consumer preferences. Comparing dynamic demand response (DDR) strategies–using next-day spot prices and emissions forecasts–with static demand response (SDR) based on historical trends showed that DDR consistently delivers higher savings and emissions reductions. Flexible loads included common household appliances (washing machine, dishwasher, tumble dryer) and EVs. Allowing load shifting throughout the whole day achieved the highest savings, mainly due to low-price nighttime hours. Based on 2021 Finnish data, households could save up to €250 per year if prioritizing financial benefits alone, or reduce up to 100 kg of CO_2 annually if focusing solely on emissions. A balanced preference offers both with moderate trade-offs, underscoring the value of dynamic, automated scheduling for households.

Secondly, the dissertation explored the diversity of consumer motivations and clustered households into three key subgroups: Adopters, Followers, and Neutrals. Based on a survey among Finnish households, roughly 17% were Adopters–tech-savvy, early adopters motivated by smart home automation. About 31% were Followers–motivated by social influence and friends' choices rather than technology itself. The remaining were Neutral–households indifferent to DR motivators. Socioeconomic factors, such as education level, income, and dwelling type, were found to significantly affect these groupings. This clustering provides useful insights for tailoring DR programs and policy outreach to specific household profiles.

Extending this, the research quantified households' WTE different flexible loads. Findings show consumers generally expect higher economic savings to justify participation, especially for heating, which requires more compensation than appliances or EVs. This contrasts with earlier literature, likely due to changing electricity prices and differences in heating systems. Younger, higher-educated consumers were more open to enrolling EVs and heating, while females and households without children showed higher WTE overall.

An extrapolation using iterative proportional fitting further refined these insights to better reflect the actual Finnish population. It found that the share of Adopters and Followers increase significantly while considering the national statistics of Finland, positioning Finland as an ideal testbed for large-scale residential DR pilots.

The impact of external shocks, such as the energy crisis caused by the war in Ukraine, was also examined. A follow-up survey conducted before and during the crisis (March and September 2022) demonstrated a significant increase in households' willingness to shift loads–from 60% to 80%. Acceptance rose across all demographics, with females and older consumers showing the greatest increases. Regional and dwelling-type disparities narrowed as well. This shows that during crises, clear communication and incentives can mobilize broad consumer participation, supporting grid stability in times of stress.

The dissertation validated an ABM framework to simulate consumer DR enrollment. This model captures both personal savings expectations and social dynamics by representing each consumer as an agent embedded in neighborhoods with social connections. By testing various contract types with differing levels of flexibility and commitment, the study highlighted seasonal and behavioral enrollment patterns. For instance, flexible monthly contracts saw peak enrollment in winter when potential savings are highest, while binding contracts showed delayed but sustained adoption. Sensitivity analyses demonstrated that factors such as the share of heat pump or PV-battery owners and expected annual savings strongly affect enrollment levels, while the direct influence of friends was less significant than anticipated.

Lastly, the dissertation explored pricing schemes for aggregators to incentivize load-shifting. Results showed that aggregators could earn profits while providing incentives, though uncertainty remains if consumers do not shift loads as expected. A Monte Carlo simulation showed reduced profits, laying groundwork for pilot implementation.

Overall, this dissertation advances the understanding of residential DR potential by bridging technical, economic, and behavioral dimensions. Its insights can inform policymakers, utilities, and DR service providers on how to design more effective, consumer-centric flexibility programs that harness diverse motivations and adapt to changing market and societal conditions.

5 Discussion and Concluding Remarks

This dissertation has advanced the understanding of residential DR by investigating the complex factors that shape consumer decision-making and enrollment behavior. As flexibility becomes critical for the sustainable transformation of the electricity system, residential consumers will play an increasingly central role. The research contributes novel insights by bridging gaps in how consumer motivations, preferences, and socioeconomic contexts affect DR participation.

First, the work highlights that consumer preferences toward DR motivators–financial, environmental, and social–are diverse and clustered into subgroups. Recognizing these differences, the research demonstrates that there is no "one-size-fits-all" solution; targeted and tailored DR programs are needed to maximize adoption and effectiveness.

Second, by quantifying consumers' willingness to engage household loads in DLC schemes, the study shows that both financial savings and CO_2 reductions drive participation. This interplay varies by subgroup, offering guidance for policymakers and aggregators to design more responsive and inclusive DR campaigns.

The dissertation also reveals that societal factors strongly shape decision-making. Using an ABM, the research simulates how social influence, neighborhood effects, and contract flexibility affect enrollment rates. These dynamics underscore the need to embed DR programs within communities, fostering positive feedback loops that sustain participation even when financial returns diminish.

Additionally, this work emphasizes that DR must evolve beyond short-term spot price arbitrage, which risks self-cannibalization through reduced price volatility. Instead, the findings support reframing DR as a lifestyle–where environmental awareness, community participation, and shared responsibility for grid stability become key motivators alongside financial incentives. Behavioral shifts during the recent energy crisis illustrate this potential.

From an aggregator's perspective, the dissertation confirms that well-designed incentive schemes can deliver mutual benefits, though uncertainty remains if consumers do not shift loads as expected. Robust strategies–including real-world pilot projects–are essential to validate these models, refine pricing structures, and build trust in DR offerings.

Future research should test the proposed frameworks in practice, incorporate more diverse market services such as frequency regulation, explore real-world price elasticities using machine learning, and close the feedback loop between models and observed behavior. Ultimately, by connecting modeling with practical deployment, future work can help embed DR as a resilient, widely accepted part of everyday life, supporting the transition to a flexible, low-carbon energy system.

References

1. H.A. Aalami, H. Pashaei-Didani, S. Nojavan, Deriving nonlinear models for incentive-based demand response programs. Int. J. Electr. Power Energy Syst. **106**, 223–231 (2019). https://doi.org/10.1016/j.ijepes.2018.10.003
2. T. Broberg, L. Persson, Is our everyday comfort for sale? preferences for demand management on the electricity market. Energy Econ. **54**, 24–32 (2016). https://doi.org/10.1016/j.eneco.2015.11.005
3. K. Christensen, Z. Ma, Y. Demazeau, B.N. Jørgensen, Agent-based modeling of climate and electricity market impact on commercial greenhouse growers' demand response adoption, in *2020 RIVF International Conference on Computing and Communication Technologies (RIVF)* (IEEE, 2020), pp 1–7. https://doi.org/10.1109/RIVF48685.2020.9140789
4. T.H. Meles, L. Ryan, Adoption of renewable home heating systems: an agent-based model of heat pumps in Ireland. Renew. Sustain. Energy Rev. **169**, 112853 (2022). https://doi.org/10.1016/j.rser.2022.112853
5. D. Muthirayan, D. Kalathil, K. Poolla, P. Varaiya, Baseline estimation and scheduling for demand response, in *2018 IEEE Conference on Decision and Control (CDC)* (IEEE, 2018), pp. 4857–4862. https://doi.org/10.1109/CDC.2018.8619236
6. P. Palensky, D. Dietrich, Demand side management: demand response, intelligent energy systems, and smart loads. IEEE Trans. Ind. Inf. **7**(3), 381–388 (2011). https://doi.org/10.1109/TII.2011.2158841
7. E. Ruokamo, M. Kopsakangas-Savolainen, T. Meriläinen, R. Svento, Towards flexible energy demand-preferences for dynamic contracts, services and emissions reductions. Energy Econ. **84**, 104522 (2019). https://doi.org/10.1016/j.eneco.2019.104522
8. A. Sridhar, S. Honkapuro, F. Ruiz, S. Annala, A. Wolff, Assessing the economic and environmental benefits of residential demand response: a finnish case study, in *2022 18th International*

Conference on the European Energy Market (EEM) (IEEE, 2022), pp. 1–6 . https://doi.org/10.1109/EEM54602.2022.9921144

9. A. Sridhar, S. Honkapuro, F. Ruiz, S. Annala, A. Wolff, The impact of an energy crisis on the residential consumers' consumption behavior based on a finish case study, in *2023 IEEE PES Innovative Smart Grid Technologies Europe (ISGT EUROPE)* (IEEE, 2023), pp. 1–5. https://doi.org/10.1109/ISGTEUROPE56780.2023.10407776

10. A. Sridhar, S. Honkapuro, F. Ruiz, J. Stoklasa, S. Annala, A. Wolff, A. Rautiainen, Nation-wide projection of motivators and consumer willingness for direct load control demand response in finland. In: 27th International Conference on Electricity Distribution (CIRED 2023) (IET, 2023), pp. 401–405. https://doi.org/10.1049/icp.2023.0328

11. A. Sridhar, S. Honkapuro, F. Ruiz, J. Stoklasa, S. Annala, A. Wolff, A. Rautiainen, Residential consumer preferences to demand response: analysis of different motivators to enroll in direct load control demand response. Energy Policy **173**, 113420 (2023). https://doi.org/10.1016/j.enpol.2023.113420

12. A. Sridhar, S. Honkapuro, F. Ruiz, J. Stoklasa, S. Annala, A. Wolff, A. Rautiainen, Toward residential flexibility-consumer willingness to enroll household loads in demand response. Appl. Energy **342**, 121204 (2023). https://doi.org/10.1016/j.apenergy.2023.121204

13. A. Sridhar, S. Honkapuro, F. Ruiz, J. Stoklasa, S. Annala, A. Wolff, Consumer enrollment in residential demand response: Implications across diverse societies, in *2024 IEEE PES Innovative Smart Grid Technologies—Asia (ISGT Asia)*, pp. 1–6 (2024). https://doi.org/10.1109/ISGTAsia61245.2024.10876367

14. A. Sridhar, S. Honkapuro, F. Ruiz, J. Stoklasa, S. Annala, A. Wolff, Residential consumer enrollment in demand response: an agent based approach. Appl. Energy **374**, 123988 (2024). https://doi.org/10.1016/j.apenergy.2024.123988

15. A. Sridhar, S. Honkapuro, F. Ruiz, B. Mohammadi-Ivatloo, S. Annala, A. Wolff, Aggregator decision analysis in residential demand response under uncertain consumer behavior. J. Clean. Product. **495**, 144997 (2025). https://doi.org/10.1016/j.jclepro.2025.144997, https://www.sciencedirect.com/science/article/pii/S0959652625003476

16. A. Sridhar, S. Honkapuro, F. Ruiz, J. Stoklasa, S. Annala, A. Wolff, Residential demand response enrollment scenarios: a geospatial case study of Finland, in *2025 21st International Conference on the European Energy Market (EEM)*, pp. 1–7. https://doi.org/10.1109/EEM64765.2025.11050084

17. K. Stenner, E.R. Frederiks, E.V. Hobman, S. Cook, Willingness to participate in direct load control: the role of consumer distrust. Appl. Energy **189**, 76–88 (2017). https://doi.org/10.1016/j.apenergy.2016.10.099

18. J. Vuelvas, F. Ruiz, Rational consumer decisions in a peak time rebate program. Electr. Power Syst. Res. **143**, 533–543 (2017). https://doi.org/10.1016/j.epsr.2016.11.001

19. S. Yilmaz, P. Cuony, C. Chanez, Prioritize your heat pump or electric vehicle? Analysing design preferences for direct load control programmes in Swiss households. Energy Res. Soc. Sci. **82**, 102319 (2021). https://doi.org/10.1016/j.erss.2021.102319

Telecommunications

Cooperative Machine Learning Methods in Distributed Systems

Bernardo Camajori Tedeschini

Abstract Cooperative machine learning is reshaping how multi-agent systems handle massive, distributed, and privacy-sensitive data streams. This chapter condenses my doctoral work on two fronts: learning, which builds shared models, and inference, which uses those models in real time. For learning, we propose graph-aware message-passing neural networks that surpass classical belief propagation in data association and joint positioning, fully decentralized federated and split schemes that protect privacy and save energy in medical and internet of things (IoT) settings, and a reinforcement framework that keeps localization accurate in highly dynamic vehicle swarms. For inference, we present a single-pass detector for instant non-line-of-sight recognition, a latent-feature fusion method that switches smoothly between standalone and cooperative static positioning, and a sampling-free Bayesian kernel that attaches trustworthy aleatoric and epistemic uncertainty to mobile tracking. Together, these contributions form a coherent toolbox that turns heterogeneous 5G/6G, robotic, and healthcare networks into reliable, low-latency cyber-physical systems.

1 Introduction

Multi-agent systems (MAS) have become a cornerstone of modern cyber-physical infrastructures [1]. From surgical imaging networks to swarms of connected automated vehicles, physically separated agents now generate orders of magnitude more

The fundamental research described in the thesis was supported, in part, by the Roberto Rocca Doctoral Fellowship awarded by Politecnico di Milano and Massachusetts Institute of Technology (MIT), by the project Centro Nazionale per la Mobilità Sostenibile (MOST), funded by the Italian Ministry of University and Research under the Piano Nazionale Ripresa Resilienza (PNRR) funding program, by the European Space Agency (ESA) Navigation Innovation and Support Program (NAVISP) Element 2 pillar, by the Horizon EU project TRUSTroke in the call HORIZON-HLTH-2022-STAYHLTH-01-two-stage under GA No. 101080564, by the National Science Foundation under Grant CNS-2148251, and by the federal agency and industry partners in the RINGS Program.

B. Camajori Tedeschini (✉)
QUALCOMM R&D, Lannion, France
e-mail: bernardo.camajori@polimi.it

C. Cappiello (ed.), *Special Topics in Information Technology*,
PoliMI SpringerBriefs, https://doi.org/10.1007/978-3-032-12359-6_10

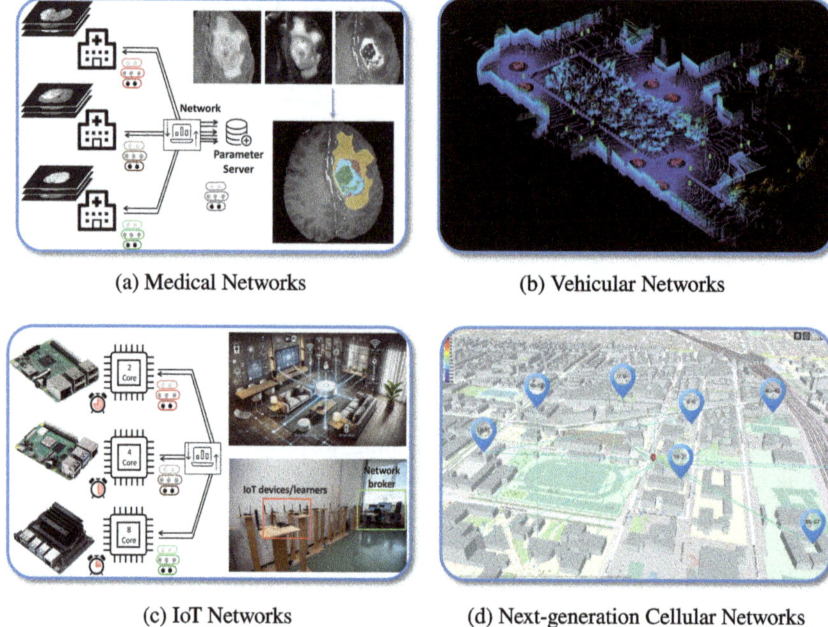

(a) Medical Networks

(b) Vehicular Networks

(c) IoT Networks

(d) Next-generation Cellular Networks

Fig. 1 Application domain of MAS

data than a single processor can digest [2]. Addressing this data influx calls for cooperative machine learning (ML) paradigms that (i) scale with the number of nodes, (ii) respect stringent latency, reliability, and privacy constraints, and (iii) remain robust when the data distribution or the network topology drifts over time. See Fig. 1 for the main application domains of MAS. For example, in a medical network [3], the focus is on learning the most accurate and reliable models for tasks like diagnosis, ensuring data privacy, and compliance with regulations. Whereas in vehicular networks [4], the emphasis is on efficiently predicting the model outcome in real-time for applications such as cooperative positioning (CP). Thus, we can distinguish between cooperative learning and inference based on their distinct roles and methodologies, each tailored to optimize different aspects of MAS.

Cooperative learning builds global models by fusing observations gathered across the graph. Centralized machine learning (C-ML) excel when high-capacity edge servers are available, whereas decentralized machine learning (D-ML)/ fully decentralized machine learning (FD-ML) and split architectures split learning (SL) safeguard sensitive data and cope with device heterogeneity [5]. Once a model is in place, cooperative inference exploits on-line collaboration to enhance mission-critical tasks such as joint non-line-of-sight (NLoS) identification, centimeter-level CP, and real-time tracking with calibrated uncertainty in next-generation cellular networks.

Despite recent progress, three key challenges persist: first, learning algorithms must remain graph-aware so that performance does not collapse on loopy, non-

Gaussian interaction graphs [6]; second, training must be both privacy-preserving and scalable when data are non-IID and connectivity is intermittent, which rules out naïve synchronous federated updates [7]; third, safety-critical applications require predictions equipped with trustworthy, real-time uncertainty estimates rather than point values alone [8].

This chapter presents the key ideas of the doctoral work into a compact narrative. We (a) augment traditional message passing algorithm (MPA) with data-driven message passing neural networks (MPNNs) for robust data association (DA)/CP; (b) design asynchronous, weighted-consensus federated learning (FL) and fully-decentralized split consensus federated learning (SCFL) to meet privacy and energy budgets; and (c) introduce a single-shot anomaly detector (deep autoencoding kernel density model (DAKDM)) and a sampling-free Bayesian framework (Bayesian bright knowledge (BBK)) that jointly quantify aleatoric and epistemic uncertainty, enabling trustworthy 5G/6G sensing.

The chapter is organized as follows. Section 2 summarizes the cooperative-learning contributions: graph-aware MPNN [9–11], privacy-preserving FL and SL [12–15], and non-stationary multi-agent reinforcement learning (MARL) [16, 17]. Section 3 details the inference pipeline for next-generation cellular sensing, covering single-shot anomaly detection [18], cooperative static positioning [19], and sampling-free Bayesian tracking [20, 21]. Finally, Sect. 4 draws the conclusions.

In addition to the mentioned contributions and articles, the research carried out during the Ph.D. has led to several other publications that have not been included as they are beyond the coverage of this thesis [22–31].

2 Cooperative Learning

2.1 Graph-Aware Learning

In this chapter, we present two works that perform cooperative learning directly on graphs. Specifically, within the framework of vehicular networks, we propose the integration and employment of MPNN into C-ML systems for the tasks of DA and CP (see Fig. 2 for a representation of the cooperative scenario). In the first paper [9, 10], the objective is to associate measurements obtained with lidar object detection models at different vehicles. To tackle the problem, we present a logical graph mapping based on the measurements, i.e., detections, and the vehicles' positions. We then associate different measurements by means of a modified MPNN model trained on edge-classification task on the logical graph. Finally, we compare the performances of the proposed approach with MPA-based algorithms under different noise conditions and graph dimensions. The results demonstrate that the proposed MPNN model effectively learns the correct associations across a range of realistic measurement

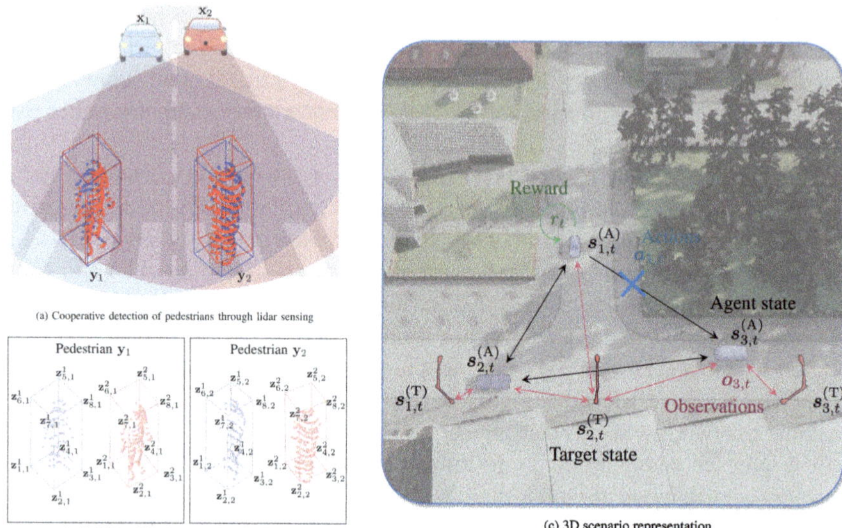

Fig. 2 **a** Cooperative scenario with vehicles detecting two pedestrians by means of lidar technology. **b** Bounding boxes extracted from the lidar point cloud with corner definition. **c** 3D representation of the scenario with three vehicles and three objects (snapshot extracted from CARLA software). Agent-to-agent communication links and agent-to-target detections are indicated with black and red arrows, respectively

conditions and generalizes well to previously unseen scenarios, including varying error statistics, noise levels, vehicle counts, and new environments.

In the second paper [11], the objective becomes performing CP in a distributed network of agents that move in the space and gather state and inter-agent measurements at each timestep. Inspired by the MPA for CP, we propose a two-block model, namely long short-term memory (LSTM)-MPNN, that employs the LSTM for next state prediction and the MPNN for measurements processing and state update. The results indicate that the developed LSTM-MPNN model surpasses the corresponding MPA in CP in both complexity and accuracy. This improvement is achieved by directly learning the state-transition probability density function (PDF) and the distributed state-update from trajectory data.

2.2 Federated and Split Learning

In this chapter, we present four works on distributed cooperative learning, namely D-ML and FD-ML. The distributed algorithms are studied in a real FL platform developed in the first paper [12] for performing privacy-preserving brain tumor segmentation in medical networks. The platform is based on the message queuing telemetry transport (MQTT) protocol, and it is flexible to different models, i.e., architectures and sizes, as well as different FL algorithms, i.e., centralized and decentralized FL. Motivated by the open issue of synchronization in FL processes, in the second paper [13] we propose guidelines for designing asynchronous parameter server (PS) orchestration under heterogeneous internet of things (IoT) devices. In particular, we tune the intervals between consecutive global model updates based on sample distributions and computational capabilities, enhancing the accuracy of the system.

Subsequently, in the third paper [14], we address the problem of non-independent and identically distributed (IID) data distributions in decentralized FL processes by proposing weighted averaged consensus (WAC) schemes applied to consensus-based FL. Specifically, we evolve the centralized federated adaptive weighting (FedAdp) method and introduce three distinct WAC schemes, named consensus-driven FedAdp (CFAdp), tailored for heterogeneous client populations. Results on real IoT devices show an improvement in both convergence and performances under both label and sample data skewness. Finally, in the last paper [15], the objective was to create a new class of FD-ML algorithms for both distributed learning and inferences under resource-constrained devices. Inspired by the recent introduction of split federated learning (SFL) algorithms, we propose a novel server-less SCFL framework that combines the advantages of both SL and consensus-based FL algorithms. SCFL is based on an innovative distributed version of MPNN, which enables privacy-preserving and fully-decentralized learning, as well as low-model complexity for IoT devices and parallel training and testing among agents.

2.3 Multi-agent Reinforcement Learning

In this chapter, we present a data-driven approach for extending the implicit cooperative positioning (ICP) framework and overcoming its main limitations due to the cyclicity of the factor graph [16, 17]. In particular, we propose a MARL algorithm, namely ICP-multi-agent proximal policy optimization (MAPPO), tailored for highly non-stationary learning where the agent network, i.e., a vehicular network, continuously varies in time. We model the problem as a decentralized-partially observable Markov decision process (Dec-POMDP) where agents aim at performing CP by exploiting exchanged measurements, comprising detection of passive objects that act as reference points to refine the predictions. The agents predict the state evolution by beliefs learning and follow a policy that dictates which links deactivate to simultaneously improve performances and achieve high communication efficiency. To solve the issue of partial observability of the state, we employ the C-ML paradigm for training, with subsequent deployment of the models for decentralized execution. Results show that this new scheme, named centralized-training and dynamic-decentralized-execution, is able to outperform the ICP algorithm when it comes to both positioning accuracy, speed of convergence and efficiency of neighbors' cooperation.

3 Cooperative Inference

3.1 Efficient Distribution Sampling for NLoS Identification

In this chapter, we present a work [18] on efficient distribution sampling for NLoS identification in next-generation cellular networks, modelling the problem as an anomaly detection task. In particular, we address the limitations of current semi-supervised learning methods in providing a precise and compact latent feature representation that does not require two-stage training and holding the entire training dataset for prediction. To this aim, we propose a DAKDM composed of an autoencoder (AE), a kernel density estimation (KDE) and a likelihood network. The AE permits to have a compact representation of the input, i.e., angle-delay channel power matrix (ADCPM), by minimizing the reconstruction error. On the contrary, the likelihood network is trained to mimic the KDE output adopting the variational inference (VI) paradigm. At inference phase, the decoder and KDE parts are discarded, and only the encoder and likelihood networks are adopted for anomaly score estimation. The base stations (BSs) are trained according to the C-ML paradigm by only employing line-of-sight (LoS) data, i.e., normal data, whereas they are tested to distinguish NLoS samples, i.e., anomalous data, from the learned LoS distribution. Comparisons with statistical and deep learning (DL) methods for anomaly detection show that the proposed DAKDM is able to have similar performances to best state-of-the-art methods while being significantly more efficient in terms of storage requirements and inference time.

3.2 Efficient Latent Features Combination for Static Positioning

In this chapter, we deal with the task of CP through next-generation BSs which aim at performing static positioning of a user equipment (UE) in an urban environment. The challenges are how to perform real-time positioning in both LoS and NLoS environments by exploiting the neighbors' output in an efficient manner. In the paper [19], we propose an AE-based model to extract an efficient non-linear representation of channel, comprising all received signal strength (RSS), time of flight (ToF), and angle of arrival (AoA) for every path. Subsequently, a NLoS identification model, trained in a supervised way, assigns an estimate of the NLoS probability. In case we are in NLoS, the latent features are used as fingerprint to perform localization with a single-BS, i.e., egocentric mode. On the contrary, in the case of LoS condition, the latent features are exchanged among BSs, carefully combined, and adopted as input in a neural network (NN) for position estimation. In the simulations, we adopted ray-tracing technology for realistic channel representation, and Simulation of Urban MObility (SUMO) software for creating realistic intelligent transportation systems (C-ITS) environment in an urban micro (UMi) environment. The results demonstrate

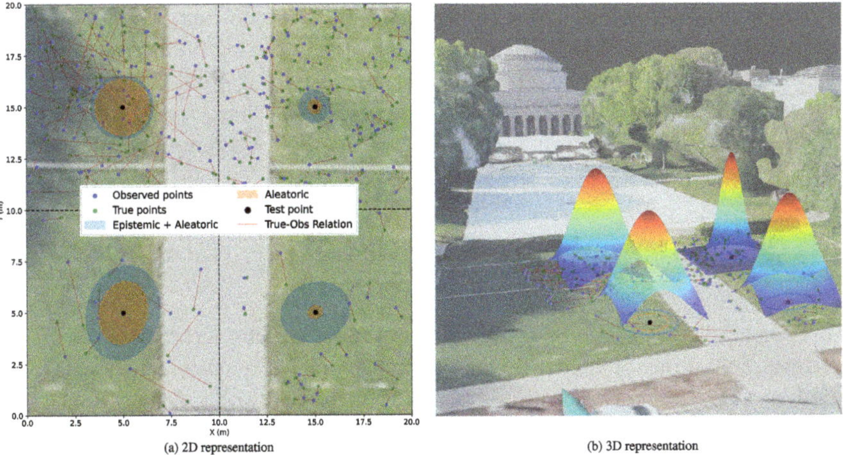

(a) 2D representation   (b) 3D representation

Fig. 3 Epistemic and aleatoric uncertainty visualization in a 3D scenario. **a** Bird's-eye view representation and **b** 3D representation obtained through Google Maps, RenderDoc, and Blender software

that the cooperative architecture particularly enhances the performance over traditional geometric algorithms, and solves the limits of single-BS predictions with DL by dynamically changing strategies based on the scenario.

3.3 Efficient Uncertainty Quantification for Mobile Positioning

In this chapter, we tackle the task of UE tracking in urban environments with next-generation cellular networks. Given the presence of high-blockage conditions, the main challenge is how to estimate in real-time the reliability of DL model predictions. In the paper [20, 21], we propose two complementary contributions to this challenge. First, we propose the integration of Bayesian neural network (BNN) into tracking filters by exploiting the predicted uncertainty as likelihood measure, which permits the coherent combination of multiple BSs' position estimates. Second, we introduce a novel BNN algorithm, namely BBK, which exploits the teacher-student paradigm to perform uncertainty quantification without the need of performing sampling procedures at inference phase (see Fig. 3 for an example of uncertainty estimation obtained in a 3D scenario). Moreover, BBK, as opposed to state-of-the-art real-time BNN methods, is able to fully evaluate the output's uncertainty by distinguishing between aleatoric and epistemic uncertainties. This enables insights behind the uncertainty prediction and can guide for more efficient sample gathering. We test the proposed BBK method with an AE-based DL model which predicts the UE position from ADCPM samples. The results indicate that the BBK approach can accurately estimate both aleatoric and epistemic uncertainties, surpassing the performances of current real-time BNN methods, particularly in out of distribution (OoD) scenarios. In terms of mobile positioning, the proposed cooperative tracking method outperforms traditional geometric tracking filters, as well as recurrent neural network (RNN) models thanks to the coherent fusion of multiple BSs predictions.

4 Concluding Remarks

This chapter showcased how cooperative machine-learning techniques can lift the intrinsic limitations of model-driven approaches in multi-agent networks. On the learning side, graph-aware message-passing neural networks enable robust data association and cooperative perception; asynchronous, privacy-preserving federated and split schemes scale training to heterogeneous devices; and a centralised-training/dynamic-execution paradigm extends reinforcement learning to non-stationary vehicular swarms. Together, these contributions provide a versatile toolbox that transforms raw, distributed data into reliable global models while respecting stringent latency, energy, and confidentiality budgets.

On the inference side, we introduced three complementary building blocks: (i) a single-shot anomaly detector that recognises NLoS conditions without costly density sampling, (ii) an adaptive latent-feature fusion strategy that switches between ego and cooperative positioning, and (iii) a sampling-free Bayesian kernel that delivers real-time trajectory estimates with calibrated aleatoric and epistemic uncertainties. Combined, they form a coherent sensing stack that attains centimetre-level accuracy and trustworthy confidence bounds in 5G/6G cellular networks. Future work will extend these methods to multi-object tracking, joint communication-sensing optimisation, and sim-to-real transfer, further advancing autonomous, cooperative cyber-physical systems.

References

1. A. Dorri, S.S. Kanhere, R. Jurdak, Multi-agent systems: A survey. IEEE Access **6**, 28573–28593 (Apr.2018)
2. Y. Cao et al., An overview of recent progress in the study of distributed multi-agent coordination. IEEE Trans. Ind. Inform. **9**(1), 427–438 (Feb.2013)
3. N. Rieke *et al.*, "The future of digital health with federated learning," *npj Digital Med.*, vol. 3, no. 1, p. 119, Sep. 2020
4. Q. Yang et al., Machine-learning-enabled cooperative perception for connected autonomous vehicles: Challenges and opportunities. IEEE Netw. **35**(3), 96–101 (May2021)
5. J. Konečný *et al.*, "Federated optimization: Distributed machine learning for on-device intelligence," *ArXiv*, Oct. 2016
6. F. Meyer et al., Message passing algorithms for scalable multitarget tracking. Proc. IEEE **106**(2), 221–259 (Feb.2018)

7. Y. Chen *et al.*, "Asynchronous online federated learning for edge devices with non-IID data," in *2020 IEEE Int. Conf. Big Data (Big Data)*, Dec. 2020, pp. 15–24

8. *Study on enhancement of 3GPP Support for 5G V2X Services*, TR 22.886 Version 16.2.0, 3rd Generation Partnership Project (3GPP), Sophia Antipolis, France, Dec. 2018

9. B. Camajori Tedeschini *et al.*, "Addressing data association by message passing over graph neural networks," in *2022 25th Int. Conf. Inf. Fusion (FUSION)*, Jul. 2022, pp. 01–07

10. B. Camajori Tedeschini *et al.*, "Cooperative lidar sensing for pedestrian detection: Data association based on message passing neural networks," *IEEE Trans. Signal Process.*, vol. 71, pp. 3028–3042, Aug. 2023

11. B. Camajori Tedeschini, M. Brambilla, and M. Nicoli, "Message passing neural network versus message passing algorithm for cooperative positioning," *IEEE Trans. Cogn. Commun. Netw.*, vol. 9, no. 6, pp. 1666–1676, Aug. 2023

12. B. Camajori Tedeschini *et al.*, "Decentralized federated learning for healthcare networks: A case study on tumor segmentation," *IEEE Access*, vol. 10, pp. 8693–8708, Jan. 2022

13. B. Camajori Tedeschini, S. Savazzi, and M. Nicoli, "A traffic model based approach to parameter server design in federated learning processes," *IEEE Commun. Lett.*, vol. 27, no. 7, pp. 1774–1778, May 2023

14. B. Camajori Tedeschini, S. Savazzi, and M. Nicoli, "Weighted consensus algorithms in distributed and federated learning," *IEEE Trans. Netw. Sci. and Eng.*, vol. 12, no. 2, pp. 1369–1382, 2024

15. B. Camajori Tedeschini, M. Brambilla, and M. Nicoli, "Split consensus federated learning: an approach for distributed training and inference," *IEEE Access*, vol. 12, pp. 119 535–119 549, Aug. 2024

16. B. Camajori Tedeschini, "Cooperative positioning with multi-agent reinforcement learning,âĿž in, et al., 27th Int. Conf. Inf. Fusion (FUSION) **2024**, 1–7 (2024)

17. B. Camajori Tedeschini *et al.*, "Multi-agent reinforcement learning for distributed cooperative positioning," *IEEE Trans. Intell. Veh.*, pp. 1–16, Oct. 2024

18. B. Camajori Tedeschini, M. Nicoli, and M. Z. Win, "On the latent space of mmWave MIMO channels for NLOS identification in 5G-advanced systems," *IEEE J. Sel. Areas Commun.*, vol. 41, no. 6, pp. 1655–1669, May 2023

19. B. Camajori Tedeschini and M. Nicoli, "Cooperative deep-learning positioning in mmWave 5G-advanced networks," *IEEE J. Sel. Areas Commun.*, vol. 41, no. 12, pp. 3799–3815, Dec. 2023

20. B. Camajori Tedeschini *et al.*, "Empowering 6G positioning and tracking with Bayesian neural networks," in *ICC 2024 - 2024 IEEE Int. Conf. Commun. (ICC)*. IEEE, Jun. 2024, pp. 1–6

21. B. Camajori Tedeschini *et al.*, "Real-time Bayesian neural networks for 6G cooperative positioning and tracking," *IEEE J. Sel. Areas Commun.*, vol. 42, no. 9, pp. 2322–2338, Aug. 2024

22. B. Camajori Tedeschini *et al.*, "A feasibility study of 5G positioning with current cellular network deployment," *Sci. Reports*, vol. 13, no. 1, Sep. 2023

23. L. Barbieri *et al.*, "Implicit vehicle positioning with cooperative lidar sensing," in *ICASSP 2023 - 2023 IEEE Int. Conf. Acoust., Speech Signal Process. (ICASSP)*, Jun. 2023, pp. 1–5, iSSN: 2379-190X

24. S. Roger et al., Deep-learning-based radio map reconstruction for V2X communications. IEEE Trans. on Veh. Technol. **73**(3), 3863–3871 (Oct.2023)

25. L. Barbieri et al., Deep learning-based cooperative LiDAR sensing for improved vehicle positioning. IEEE Trans. Signal Process. **72**, 1666–1682 (Mar.2024)

26. U. Milasheuski *et al.*, "On the impact of data heterogeneity in federated learning environments with application to healthcare networks," in *IEEE Conf. Artif. Intell.* IEEE, Jun. 2024, pp. 1017–1023

27. L. Italiano *et al.*, "Pedestrian positioning in urban environments with 5G technology," in *IEEE Mediterranean Commun. and Comput. Netw. Conf.* IEEE, Jun. 2024, pp. 1–6

28. L. Italiano et al., A tutorial on 5G positioning. IEEE Commun. Surveys & Tuts **27**(3), 1488–1535 (Aug.2025)

29. M. Brambilla *et al.*, "Integration of 5G and GNSS technologies for enhanced positioning: an experimental study," *IEEE Open J. of the Commun. Soc.*, vol. 5, pp. 7197–7215, Nov. 2024
30. N. Schatz *et al.*, "Location verification in next-generation non-terrestrial networks," in *IEEE Military Commun. Conf.* IEEE, Nov. 2024, pp. 1–6
31. J. C. Morrison *et al.*, "Sidelink-enabled cooperative localization for xG non-terrestrial networks," in *IEEE Military Commun. Conf.* IEEE, Nov. 2024, pp. 1–6

Data-Driven Techniques for Speech and Multimodal Deepfake Detection

Davide Salvi⊙

Abstract Recent advancements in deep learning and generative models have simplified the creation and manipulation of synthetic media. Today, even inexperienced users can produce highly realistic content with minimal effort. While these technologies offer exciting opportunities, they also pose serious risks. When misused, they can facilitate fraud, blackmail, and the spread of disinformation. An example of this phenomenon is deepfakes, synthetic multimedia content generated through deep learning techniques that depict individuals in actions and behaviors that do not belong to them. Using only a few images or an audio recording of a target victim, an attacker can utilize deepfake technology to produce synthetic data that impersonates the victim and discredits their reputation. Detecting such content is essential to prevent misuse. This chapter addresses the problem of deepfake detection, beginning with a monomodal focus on synthetic speech and then extending the analysis to audio-video multimodal deepfakes. We propose multiple detection methods and discuss broader solutions to related challenges. We view this work as a foundational but meaningful step forward in multimedia forensics. While the results are encouraging, the landscape is evolving rapidly, with emerging threats demanding continuous innovation. We believe our findings can support future research and help strengthen defenses against synthetic media misuse.

1 Introduction

Nowadays, creating and sharing multimedia content has become increasingly easy thanks to rapid advances in consumer electronics, storage capacity, internet bandwidth, and computational power. High-quality photos, videos, and audio can now be captured, edited, and globally shared using nothing more than a smartphone. As a result, the nature of online content has shifted dramatically, moving from static

D. Salvi (✉)
Politecnico di Milano, Dipartimento di Elettronica, Informazione, e Bioingegneria (DEIB), Milan, Italy
e-mail: davide.salvi@polimi.it

C. Cappiello (ed.), *Special Topics in Information Technology*,
PoliMI SpringerBriefs, https://doi.org/10.1007/978-3-032-12359-6_11

images to immersive, high-resolution videos, dominating social media platforms, which increasingly prioritize entertainment over traditional photo sharing.

In parallel with the rise of real media, synthetic content has proliferated. Powered by advances in signal processing and deep learning, particularly models such as Variational Autoencoders (VAEs), Generative Adversarial Networks (GANs), and diffusion models, realistic synthetic media can now be generated with unprecedented ease and fidelity. Tools like ChatGPT, DALL-E, Sora, and ElevenLabs can produce synthetic text, images, video, and speech that are often indistinguishable from authentic content. While these technologies present valuable opportunities for education, accessibility, and human-computer interaction, they also pose significant threats, especially when exploited for malicious purposes.

An example in this regard is deepfakes, synthetic multimedia content generated through deep learning techniques that depict individuals in actions and behaviors that do not belong to them [1, 2]. Deepfakes can be created with only a brief recording or a single image of the target, and can be weaponized to spread disinformation, damage reputations, or perpetrate fraud and extortion. The threat is not merely hypothetical: estimates suggest that the volume of deepfake content is doubling every six months, with the vast majority intended for harmful use. As such, the development of reliable and scalable methods able to detect such content has become a critical priority.

In this chapter, we consider the problem of deepfake detection and tackle it using a multimodal approach, simultaneously analyzing different content modalities to expose inconsistencies that may elude unimodal detectors. By leveraging inter-modal coherence, we aim to enhance detection robustness and resilience to adversarial techniques.

As the effectiveness of multimodal systems fundamentally depends on the quality of their individual components, we begin our analysis by focusing on audio forensics, a relatively underexplored domain compared to visual deepfake detection. As a matter of fact, weak performance in any single modality would compromise the accuracy of the entire multimodal pipeline.

First, we introduce several speech deepfake detection strategies, combining traditional signal processing with modern deep learning techniques to capitalize on their complementary strengths. Then, in the latest part of the chapter, we extend these insights to multimodal detection, proposing novel methods to exploit cross-modal consistency at a semantic level. Rather than relying on low-level generator-specific artifacts, we emphasize high-level features such as prosody, emotion, and speaker identity, which enable generalization across models, speakers, and datasets.

Our goal is to build detectors that are robust, adaptable, and capable of handling the growing complexity of synthetic media, contributing to the advancement of multimedia forensics. The content of this chapter summarizes a portion of the research conducted during my Ph.D., as documented in my dissertation [11], and further detailed in the associated publications [5, 10, 15, 19, 21–23].

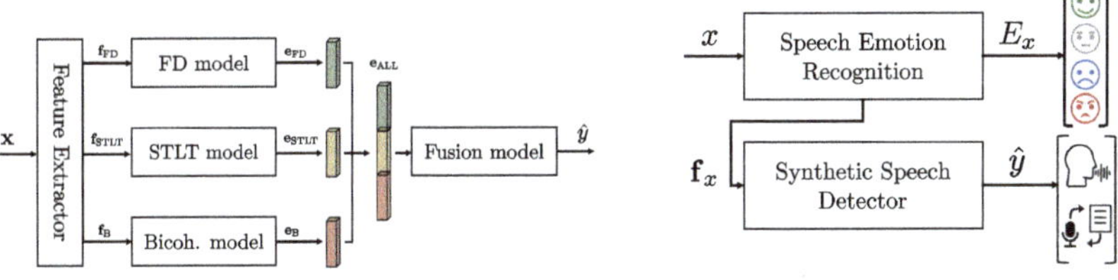

(a) Low-level feature-based detector.   (b) High-level feature-based detector.

Fig. 1 Pipelines of the proposed speech deepfake detection systems

2 Speech Deepfake Detection

The speech deepfake detection problem is formally defined as a binary classification task. Given a speech signal $\mathbf{x}$, the goal is to develop a detector $\mathcal{D}$ that estimates the probability $\hat{y} = \mathcal{D}(\mathbf{x})$ that the signal is synthetic ($y = 1$) or authentic ($y = 0$).

2.1 Detection via Low and High-Level Features

We propose two complementary detection strategies to tackle the speech deepfake detection task:

1. **Low-level feature analysis**, based on signal processing techniques that expose artifacts introduced during speech synthesis [7, 8].
2. **High-level feature analysis**, which targets semantic aspects of speech that are more difficult for generative models to replicate, such as prosody, speaker identity, and emotional expression [3, 4].

Figure 1 illustrates the pipelines for both approaches.

Each approach is motivated by the observation that synthetic speech generation systems tend to excel at mimicking low-level signal characteristics but struggle with replicating more complex nuances. For this reason, we can exploit these specific nuances to discriminate between real and fake speech signals. By combining two orthogonal perspectives, such as low and high-level feature analysis, we can build more robust and generalizable detectors.

Low-level approaches focus on statistical and spectral properties of the audio signal. While effective, traditional methods based on this setup may generalize poorly across synthesis models or under realistic distortions like noise or compression, as they focus on aspects that are too specific and, therefore, restricted. To address this limitation, we propose a fused method that integrates three distinct feature sets, each targeting different artifacts. The underlying idea is that the intra-features analyzes can be exploited to improve the robustness of the detector. The feature sets we consider are *Frequency Distribution features*, which measure deviations from the generalized

Benford's law applied to MFCC coefficients, *Short-Term Long-Term features*, that model the speech signal as a multi-order autoregressive process, detecting irregular dynamics not typical of human speech and *Bicoherence Features*, which capture higher-order bispectral correlations often present in synthesized signals but absent in natural speech.

These feature sets are fused and processed by a deep learning classifier, which proved to be robust to generalization over unseen data and against post-processing techniques that may hinder some traces left by the speech generators.

On the other hand, **high-level approaches** aim to detect forgeries by examining the semantic properties of speech, leveraging the idea that these aspects are harder to replicate faithfully using current synthesis models.

We introduce two different detectors. The first one analyzes the emotional content of speech and uses it to detect text-to-speech (TTS) data, which often lacks natural emotional variation. The second detector extends the first method by incorporating two additional aspects: speaker identity and prosody. These are extracted using transfer learning from models trained on speaker verification and prosody modeling tasks. Two distinct embeddings, capturing speaker identity and prosodic style, are extracted, concatenated, and fed into a lightweight binary classifier. This method generalizes across both TTS and voice conversion (VC) forgeries.

We evaluated the proposed low- and high-level strategies on diverse datasets and setups, demonstrating that both approaches perform well under clean and degraded conditions (e.g., compression, noise) and can be used to detect speech deepfakes in a real-world environment. The choice between the two methods depends on the use case, available data, and computational constraints. While no method currently offers universal reliability across all synthesis techniques and conditions, combining orthogonal detection cues is a promising direction for building more versatile and resilient forensic tools. By developing systems that exploit both signal-level and semantic inconsistencies, we move closer to a more comprehensive defense against the misuse of synthetic speech.

2.2 Reliability Estimation for Speech Deepfake Detection

One of the primary issues related to the use of speech deepfake detectors in real-world conditions is their low generalization capability. While many detectors show excellent performance under controlled conditions, their accuracy often drops when tested on data significantly different from the one seen during training. This poses a problem because when we evaluate an audio track using a detector, we receive an output score regardless of the reliability of the prediction, leaving us uncertain about the trustworthiness of the obtained result. In this analysis [14], we propose a classifier that can be used in parallel with a speech deepfake detector, which predicts the confidence level with which the detector assigns an authenticity score to a track under analysis. In other words, we develop a reliability estimator that assesses whether it is appropriate to input a specific audio track into a given detector. Our goal is to perform the detection process only when we are confident that the obtained score is reliable, avoiding providing misleading results. Using a simple, lightweight, dense network, the presented approach increases the detection accuracy of the model on the considered dataset and proves excellent generalization capabilities on unseen data.

2.3 Explainability in Speech Deepfake Detection

Another persistent limitation of current speech deepfake detectors is their lack of interpretability. Due to their data-driven nature, they often act like "black boxes", and we have no clue about the factors that drive their predictions. In this analysis [12, 16], we tackle the problem of explainable AI (XAI) in synthetic speech detection to understand which critical elements in a speech track influence the detectors' predictions. Our results suggest that the most relevant artifacts of synthetic speech reside in specific frequency bands. Based on this, we show how focusing only on these bands can improve the accuracy of the detection process. Additionally, as some of these bands do not include speech content, we explore the feasibility of conducting synthetic speech detection by analyzing only the background component of the signal, disregarding its verbal content. Our findings provide valuable insights for developing new speech deepfake detectors and their interpretability, together with some considerations on the existing work in the audio forensics field.

2.4 Synthetic Speech Attribution

Building on our work in speech deepfake detection, we extend our investigation to the task of attribution: the process of identifying the specific technique or model used to generate or manipulate a synthetic speech signal. While detection focuses on determining whether a signal is real or fake, attribution aims to uncover the origin of the forgery, offering finer-grained insight into the nature of the manipulation. In this study [9, 13, 17], we repurpose and adapt a set of detection models for the attribution task, evaluating their ability to differentiate among various speech synthesis methods. This allows us to assess both the versatility of existing detection approaches and the semantic distance between detection and attribution tasks. We conduct experiments in both closed-set and open-set settings and benchmark performance against a state-of-the-art attribution baseline. The results offer valuable insights into the transferability of detection techniques and the challenges specific to attribution in the context of synthetic speech forensics.

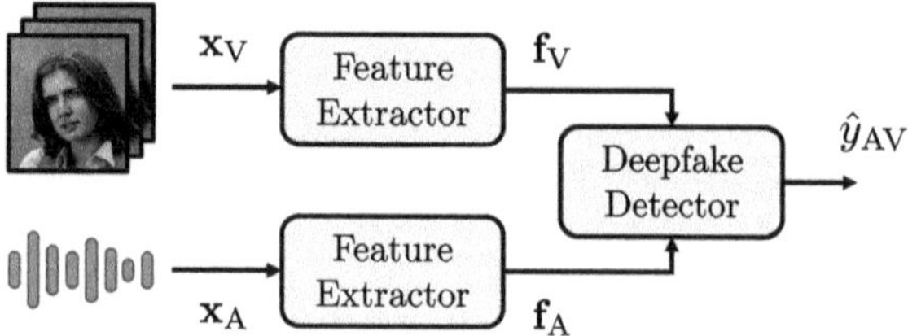

Fig. 2 General pipeline for multimodal deepfake detection

3 Multimodal Deepfake Detection

As deepfake technology evolves, the challenge of detecting forgeries is no longer limited to individual modalities like audio or video. Increasingly, synthetic content combines multiple data streams, typically audio-visual, raising the need for multimodal deepfake detection systems. In this analysis, we extend the detection problem from the monomodal to the multimodal domain and explore two complementary strategies: one based on low-level signal features, and another grounded in high-level semantic information.

This expansion poses unique challenges, such as defining effective fusion strategies across modalities and dealing with the limited availability of labeled multimodal datasets. To address these, we investigate both feature-level fusion techniques and training paradigms that rely solely on monomodal data.

Formally, let $\mathbf{x}_{AV}$ be an audio-visual signal composed of a facial video track $\mathbf{x}_V$ and a speech audio track $\mathbf{x}_A$. Each track can be either authentic ($y = 0$) or synthetic ($y = 1$). We define the label for the combined signal as: $y_{AV} = y_A \vee y_V$, where $\vee$ is the logical OR operator, indicating that the entire signal is considered fake if at least one of its modalities has been manipulated. The goal is to develop a detection model $\mathcal{D}$ that outputs a probability $\hat{y}_{AV} \in [0, 1]$ estimating the likelihood that $\mathbf{x}_{AV}$ is a deepfake, as depicted in Fig. 2.

The first approach to multimodal detection builds on **low-level features** extracted independently from audio and video signals [18, 20]. We use two modality-specific neural networks to derive features from each stream, which are then fused using different strategies to form a joint representation.

We analyze three fusion strategies, early fusion, late fusion, and intermediate fusion, evaluating their relative strengths. Among these, early fusion, where audio and video features are combined at the input stage of the classifier, proves most effective. This approach allows a deep neural network to learn cross-modal relationships from the outset, enhancing performance and robustness.

A central focus of our work is data efficiency: we explore the feasibility of training a multimodal detector using only monomodal data, a practical necessity given the scarcity of well-annotated multimodal deepfake datasets. Our findings suggest that this approach is viable, offering useful guidance for deploying multimodal detection systems in real-world environments where data limitations are common.

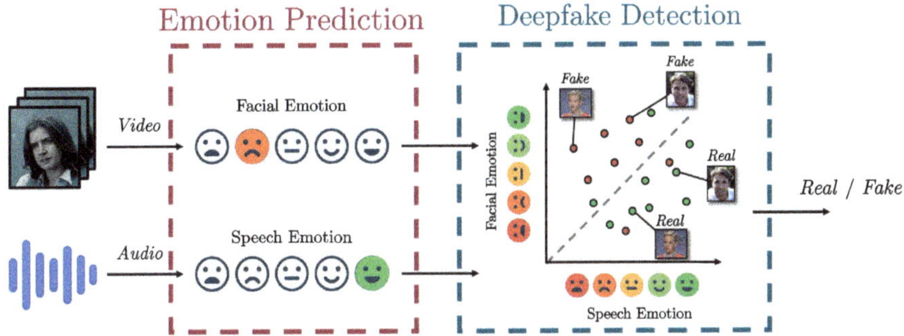

Fig. 3 Pipeline of the proposed system for multimodal deepfake detection based on emotional consistency

Building on the success of semantic-based detection for speech, we extend this strategy to the multimodal setting by focusing on **high-level features** such as emotional consistency [6]. While state-of-the-art deepfake generators can convincingly replicate low-level audio and video characteristics, they often struggle to maintain coherent emotional expression across modalities.

Our hypothesis is that inconsistencies in emotional cues, particularly between facial expressions and vocal tone, can signal manipulation. To test this, we propose a novel approach based on the valence-arousal model of emotion, a continuous two-dimensional representation where valence indicates emotional positivity and arousal reflects intensity, following the pipeline depicted in Fig. 3.

Given an audio-visual signal $\mathbf{x}_{AV}$, we extract both facial and audio features, estimate the temporal evolution of valence and arousal for each modality using LSTM-based models, and use these emotional trajectories as input to a supervised classifier. The model learns to identify discrepancies in emotional dynamics that are characteristic of deepfakes.

We evaluate our method on a SOTA dataset, focusing on cases where both modalities have been manipulated. Results show that deepfakes exhibit unnatural emotional transitions, particularly when the generation process does not explicitly synchronize affective content. Our system successfully exploits these artifacts, achieving strong detection performance and providing interpretable cues for forensic analysis.

4 Conclusions

In this chapter, we explored the problem of deepfake detection across both monomodal and multimodal scenarios, with a particular emphasis on synthetic speech and audio-visual content. We proposed a range of detection methods that combine low-level signal features with high-level semantic analysis, and we addressed auxiliary challenges such as generalization, explainability, reliability estimation, and attribution.

Our results show that combining orthogonal cues, such as signal-level artifacts and semantic inconsistencies, substantially improves detection robustness. In the monomodal case, we demonstrated that both traditional signal processing and deep learning can be effectively integrated to identify subtle traces left by speech synthesis systems. High-level features, such as emotion, prosody, and speaker identity, provided additional discriminative power and better generalization across different synthesis techniques.

In the multimodal setting, we showed that leveraging both audio and visual streams leads to significantly stronger detection performance compared to single-modality approaches. Furthermore, we demonstrated that it is possible to train multimodal detectors using only monomodal data, offering a practical solution in scenarios where comprehensive datasets are unavailable.

As deepfake generation techniques continue to evolve, we emphasize that no single detection method will suffice. Instead, the future of multimedia forensics lies in the development of flexible, modular toolsets capable of adapting to new threats. By combining diverse features, learning paradigms, and modalities, and by focusing not only on detection but also on understanding and explaining model behavior, we move closer to building resilient systems that can protect and prevent against the growing misuse of synthetic media.

References

1. I. Amerini, Mauro Barni, S. Battiato, P. Bestagini, G. Boato, T. Sari Bonaventura, V. Bruni, R. Caldelli, F. De Natale, R. De Nicola et al., Deepfake media forensics: state of the art and challenges ahead, in *International Workshop on Safeguarding Social Networks (SAFE-SN)* (2024)
2. I. Amerini, M. Barni, S. Battiato, P. Bestagini, G. Boato, V. Bruni, R. Caldelli, F. De Natale, R. De Nicola, L. Guarnera et al., Deepfake media forensics: status and future challenges. J. Imaging **11**(3), 73 (2025)
3. L. Attorresi, D. Salvi, C. Borrelli, P. Bestagini, S. Tubaro, Combining automatic speaker verification and prosody analysis for synthetic speech detection, in *International Conference on Pattern Recognition (ICPR)* (2022)
4. E. Conti, D. Salvi, C. Borrelli, B. Hosler, P. Bestagini, F. Antonacci, A. Sarti, M.C. Stamm, S. Tubaro, Deepfake speech detection through emotion recognition: a semantic approach, in *IEEE International Conference on Acoustics, Speech and Signal Processing (ICASSP)* (2022)
5. M. Gohari, D. Salvi, P. Bestagini, N. Adami, Audio features investigation for singing voice deepfake detection, in *IEEE International Conference on Acoustics, Speech and Signal Processing (ICASSP)* (2025)
6. B. Hosler, D. Salvi, A. Murray, F. Antonacci, P. Bestagini, S. Tubaro, M.C. Stamm, Do deepfakes feel emotions? A semantic approach to detecting deepfakes via emotional inconsistencies, in *IEEE/CVF Conference on Computer Vision and Pattern Recognition Workshops (CVPRW)* (2021)
7. D. Mari, D. Salvi, P. Bestagini, S. Milani, All-for-One and One-For-All: deep learning-based feature fusion for Synthetic Speech Detection, in *European Conference on Machine Learning and Knowledge Discovery in Databases Workshops (ECML PKDD)* (2023)

8. V. Negroni, D. Salvi, P. Bestagini, S. Tubaro, Analyzing the impact of splicing artifacts in partially fake speech signals. *ASVspoof 2024* (2024)
9. V. Negroni, D. Salvi, P. Bestagini, S. Tubaro, Source verification for speech deepfakes. Interspeech (2025)
10. V. Negroni, D. Salvi, A.I. Mezza, P. Bestagini, S. Tubaro, Leveraging mixture of experts for improved speech deepfake detection, in *IEEE International Conference on Acoustics, Speech and Signal Processing (ICASSP)* (2025)
11. D. Salvi, Data-driven techniques for speech and multimodal deepfake detection. *Ph.D. thesis, Politecnico di Milano*, (2024)
12. D. Salvi, T.S. Balcha, P. Bestagini, S. Tubaro, Listening between the lines: synthetic speech detection disregarding verbal content, in *IEEE International Conference on Acoustics, Speech and Signal Processing Workshops (ICASSPW)* (2024)
13. D. Salvi, P. Bestagini, S. Tubaro, Exploring the synthetic speech attribution problem through data-driven detectors, in *IEEE International Workshop on Information Forensics and Security (WIFS)* (2022)
14. D. Salvi, P. Bestagini, S. Tubaro, Reliability estimation for synthetic speech detection, in *IEEE International Conference on Acoustics, Speech and Signal Processing (ICASSP)* (2023)
15. D. Salvi, P. Bestagini, S. Tubaro, Synthetic speech detection through audio folding, in *ACM International Workshop on Multimedia AI against Disinformation (MAD)* (2023)
16. D. Salvi, P. Bestagini, S. Tubaro, Towards frequency band explainability in synthetic speech detection, in *European Signal Processing Conference (EUSIPCO)* (2023)
17. D. Salvi, C. Borrelli, P. Bestagini, F. Antonacci, M. Stamm, L. Marcenaro, A. Majumdar, Synthetic speech attribution: highlights from the IEEE signal processing cup 2022 student competition [SP Competitions]. IEEE Signal Process. Mag. **40**(6), 92–98 (2023)
18. D. Salvi, B. Hosler, P. Bestagini, M.C. Stamm, S. Tubaro, TIMIT-TTS: a text-to-speech dataset for multimodal synthetic media detection. IEEE Access **11**, 50851–50866 (2023)
19. D. Salvi, *Daniele Ugo Leonzio, Antonio Giganti, Claudio Eutizi, Sara Mandelli, Paolo Bestagini, and Stefano Tubaro* (A dataset for smartphone model identification from audio recordings. IEEE Access, Poliphone, 2025)
20. D. Salvi, H. Liu, S. Mandelli, P. Bestagini, W. Zhou, W. Zhang, S. Tubaro, A robust approach to multimodal deepfake detection. J. Imaging **9**(6), 122 (2023)
21. D. Salvi, V. Negroni, L. Bondi, P. Bestagini, S. Tubaro, Freeze and learn: continual learning with selective freezing for speech deepfake detection, in *IEEE International Conference on Acoustics, Speech and Signal Processing (ICASSP)* (2025)
22. D. Salvi, V. Negroni, S. Mandelli, P. Bestagini, S. Tubaro, Phoneme-Level analysis for person-of-interest speech deepfake detection, in *IEEE International Conference on Computer Vision Workshops (ICCVW)* (2025)
23. A.K.S. Yadav, K. Bhagtani, D. Salvi, P. Bestagini, E.J. Delp, FairSSD: understanding bias in synthetic speech detectors. In: *IEEE/CVF Conference on Computer Vision and Pattern Recognition Workshops (CVPRW)* (2024)

Green, Resilient, and Secure Next-Generation Optical Networks

Qiaolun Zhang

Abstract Optical networks represent the essential backbone for various communication systems, such as long-haul, metro, data center networks, etc. As these networks face surging volumes of highly sensitive data, it is crucial for future optical networks to efficiently accommodate rising traffic demands as well as to be resilient against network failures and secure against attackers. We aim to design resource-allocation algorithms to improve the energy efficiency, resiliency, and security of future optical networks as follows: (1) Enhance energy efficiency using novel transmission technologies. We have first investigated how to reduce energy consumption using emerging ZR/ZR+ pluggable optics, and then we have quantified the cost and power consumption of a new monitoring technique, called power profile monitoring on a network scale. (2) Improve network resilience with proactive and reactive solutions. We have investigated proactive solutions for virtual network mapping against double-link failures and reactive solutions to provide swift network recovery for future optical networks under massive failures. (3) Enhance network security with quantum technologies. We have investigated novel resource allocation algorithms for QKD networks to improve resource efficiency. Besides, we have investigated entanglement routing problems for quantum networks, which are essential for quantum applications like QKD.

1 Introduction

Future optical networks represent the essential backbone for various communication systems, such as long-haul, metro, and data center networks, etc. [1]. As future optical networks will have to handle a dramatic increase in volumes of highly sensitive data, it is crucial for future optical networks to energy-efficiently accommodate rising traffic demands as well as to be resilient to failures and secure against data loss or leakage. Specifically, the current communication systems already contribute

Q. Zhang (✉)
Department of Electronics, Information and Bioengineering, Politecnico di Milano, Milano, Italy
e-mail: qiaolun.zhang@polimi.it

© The Author(s) 2026
C. Cappiello (ed.), *Special Topics in Information Technology*,
PoliMI SpringerBriefs, https://doi.org/10.1007/978-3-032-12359-6_12

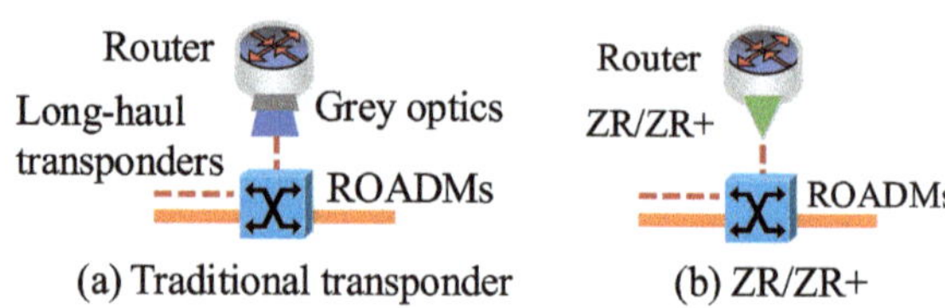

Fig. 1 Illustration of different transceivers

approximately 2–3% of global energy consumption, and the energy consumption of the future networks will increase with the ever-growing traffic demands. It is vital to develop sustainable solutions for future optical networks that reduce energy consumption. Furthermore, the future optical networks serve as an essential component for future networks such as Sixth Generation (6G) networks, which will serve various services such as autonomous driving and remote medicine. These services require developing proposals to ensure uninterrupted service during network failures (e.g., due to natural disasters). In the meantime, the data of these services contains various sensitive information. With the development of quantum technologies, quantum computers pose new threats to future optical networks by compromising traditional cryptosystems [2]. It is important to develop effective countermeasures against potential quantum attacks. Thus, we investigate the energy efficiency, resiliency, and security of future optical networks.

2 Energy Efficiency of Future Optical Networks

2.1 Power Consumption Analysis for IPoWDM Network with ZR/ZR+

Background and Motivation

Recently, ZR/ZR+ coherent transmission has attracted growing interest from vendors like Nokia [3] and Infinera for lowering transceiver cost and energy use. These advances enable architectural changes in IP-over-WDM (IPoWDM) networks to further reduce power consumption. Transparent architectures, which bypass intermediate nodes, have long been considered more energy-efficient than opaque ones. ZR/ZR+, a new type of transceiver, can connect directly to routers Fig. 1. Meanwhile, low-cost, low-power silicon technologies are reviving interest in opaque networks, which benefit from shorter transmission distances, electrical grooming, and relaxed spectrum constraints. As a result, it is crucial to reassess the energy advantage of transparent architectures. This study quantifies and compares the power consumption of IPoWDM architectures using ZR/ZR+ versus long-haul muxponders.

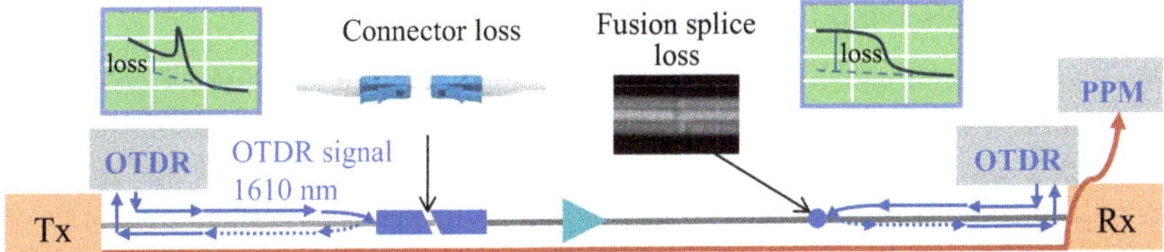

Fig. 2 Illustration of Monitoring with PPM and OTDR

Proposed Solution and Contribution

To evaluate the performance of different network architectures, we conduct a power consumption analysis for IPoWDM networks with ZR/ZR+ [4]. First, we propose a pragmatic power consumption model for different optical node architectures, considering the state-of-the-art power consumption of both IP-layer and optical-layer devices. Then, to obtain the routing for evaluating power consumption, we develop a Compact Auxiliary-Graph-based Network-Design (CAG-ND) algorithm for the Routing, Modulation format, and Spectrum Assignment problem. The proposed algorithm is extensible to all the different IPoWDM network architectures considered in this study. Finally, we conduct a sensitivity analysis to evaluate the impact of reducing power consumption in IP routers and ZR/ZR+ on various IPoWDM architectures with technology advances or adoption of devices from different vendors.

2.2 Cost and Power-Consumption Analysis for Power Profile Monitoring

Background and Motivation

Network monitoring is essential to collect comprehensive data on signal quality in optical networks. As deploying large amounts of monitoring equipment results in elevated cost and power consumption, novel low-cost monitoring methods are continuously being investigated. A new technique called *Power Profile Monitoring* (PPM) has recently gained traction thanks to its ability to monitor an entire lightpath using a single post-processing unit at the lightpath receiver. PPM does not require deploying an individual monitor for each span, as in the traditional monitoring technique using *Optical Time-Domain Reflectometer* (OTDR) as shown in Fig. 2. Instead, PPM only requires one monitor per optical line. PPM and OTDR have different monitoring applications, hence they can be considered either alternative or complementary techniques according to the targeted monitoring capabilities to be implemented in the network. In this work, we aim to quantify the cost and power consumption of PPM (using OTDR as a baseline reference), as this analysis can provide guidelines for the implementation and deployment of PPM.

Proposed Solution and Contribution

We conduct a comprehensive cost and power-consumption analysis for power profile monitoring [5]. Specifically, we are the first, to the best of our knowledge, to investigate the problem of optimized monitoring placement (OMP) and quantitatively compare the cost and power consumption of PPM and OTDR. We first prove the NP-hardness of the OMP problem and formulate an Integer Linear Programming (ILP) model for it. Moreover, to address the scalability issue of ILP, we propose an efficient heuristic algorithm that can optimize the placement of monitoring components. We provide extensive illustrative numerical evaluations to compare the cost and power consumption of PPM to OTDR. This evaluation provides guidelines for a network-wide deployment of PPM that is more cost-effective and energy-efficient than OTDR.

3 Resiliency of Future Optical Networks

3.1 Capacity Sharing for Survivable Virtual Network Mapping Under Double-Link Failures

Background and Motivation

Network slicing supports diverse services on shared infrastructure by allocating resources to virtual networks (VNs). However, it raises survivability concerns, as the failure of a single physical link can impact multiple co-located VNs, making resilience to multiple failures essential for ultra-reliable services. This work addresses the Survivable Virtual Network Mapping (SVNM) problem under double-link failures [6]. While ensuring that no two-link failure disconnects any virtual node in a VN guarantees survivability, it often requires excessive spare capacity. To reduce redundancy, we aim to improve survivability by enabling spare capacity sharing across VNs.

Proposed Solution and Contribution

We develop a capacity sharing solution for SVNM under double-link failures as follows [7]. Specifically, we propose, for the first time to the best of our knowledge, how to provide SVNM against double-link failures with inter-VN capacity sharing and devised two techniques, namely *SVNM with inter-VN capacity Sharing (SINC)* and *SVNM with inter-VN capacity Sharing and Spare Slice Sharing (SINC+)*. We first formulate a set of Integer Linear Programming (ILP) models for different SVNM scenarios, which are extensible to all the approaches with different combinations of capacity sharing and a shared spare slice. We propose a scalable heuristic algorithm that provides near-optimal (less than 2% optimality gap) solutions with a significantly shorter execution time compared to the ILP-based solution. The results show that our proposed solutions significantly improve the survivability of VNs with a small amount of additional resources compared to SVNM against single-link failures.

3.2 Progressive Slice Recovery with Guaranteed Connectivity After Massive Failures

Background and Motivation

In presence of multiple failures affecting their network infrastructure [8], operators are faced with the Progressive Network Recovery (PNR) problem, i.e., deciding the best sequence of repairs during recovery. With incoming deployments of 5G networks, PNR must evolve to incorporate new recovery opportunities offered by network slicing. In this study, we introduce the new problem of Progressive Slice Recovery (PSR), which is addressed with eight different strategies, i.e., allowing or not to change slice embedding during the recovery, and/or by enforcing different versions of slice connectivity. Specifically, we consider reachability among network nodes (network connectivity, NC) and reachability of data centers (content connectivity, CC). Since CC does not require all the nodes to be connected as NC, guaranteeing CC requires less resources compared to NC. Although guaranteeing CC may lead to service degradation, CC can still be very beneficial for disaster relief with the increasing content-centric communication paradigm.

Proposed Solution and Contribution

To address re-embedding limitations of the PSR problem, a series of on-demand progressive recovery strategies are proposed, which significantly optimize the recovery outcome after massive failures with a customized tradeoff between the cost of disruption time and slice connectivity [9]. To guarantee the provision of content-based service in 5G, we propose to take the number of slices with guaranteed connectivity constraints as one of the optimization objectives to recover slice nodes and links, which is essential to accelerate the recovery of slices. A scalable solving approach based on an auxiliary-graph-based column generation algorithm is proposed for the PSR, which obtains the recovery sequence of the substrate network in polynomial time and determines efficient re-embedding with guaranteed connectivity constraints.

4 Security of Future Optical Networks

4.1 Routing, Channel, Key-Rate and Time-Slot Assignment for QKD

Background and Motivation

To mitigate attacks from quantum computers, QKD offers a promising solution by enabling the secure exchange of keys through quantum physics principles, ensuring Information-Theoretic Security (ITS). However, QKD networks face challenges like low key rates due to factors such as fiber attenuation, the inability to amplify quantum signals, and other physical limitations [10]. The first work aims to propose a novel resource allocation algorithm for QKD networks with different settings of trusted relay (TR) and optical bypass (OB), where TR can be used to increase the key rate while OB can be used to reduce the number of QKD modules (i.e., transceivers in QKD networks). Moreover, the cache (quantum key pool, QKP) in QKD networks can be utilized to increase the performance of QKD networks under varying key demands. Specifically, unused keys generated in low-load periods can be stored in QKP and later used during high-load periods. The goal of this work is to design resource-efficient algorithms for QKD networks, utilizing QKP, across various network settings.

Proposed Solution and Contribution

We define and solve the novel Routing, Channel, Key-rate and Time-slot Assignment (RCKTA) problem to achieve resource-efficient QKD networking with QKP [11]. Specifically, we classify different network settings with optical bypass and trusted relay and prove that for all network settings, the RCKTA problem is NP-hard. We formulate a Mixed Integer Linear Programming (MILP) model for all network settings of the RCKTA problem that incorporates the limitations of the secret key rate. Our formulation accounts for the possibility of building QKD paths with not only quantum channels, but also virtual links with QKP. We propose a scalable and near-optimal heuristic algorithm for the RCKTA problem, which reduces the execution time of establishing QKD paths significantly. Numerical results show that allowing both trusted relay and optical bypass can achieve the highest acceptance ratio at the cost of only a few additional QKD modules.

4.2 Link Configuration for Entanglement Routing

Background and Motivation

This work addresses the challenge of securing future optical networks by proposing a resource allocation algorithm for distributing entangled states in quantum networks. Efficient generation and distribution of high-fidelity entanglement are essential for enabling applications such as quantum key distribution (QKD) and quantum teleportation. To establish entanglement between non-adjacent nodes, intermediate nodes perform entanglement swapping on adjacent links, forming the basis of the entanglement routing (ER) problem. While traditional ER assumes fixed-fidelity links, recent advances show that quantum links can support configurable combinations of fidelity and entanglement rate [12]. This flexibility allows more adaptive resource allocation but introduces the challenge of selecting link configurations that meet application-specific fidelity requirements. This work aims to optimize link configurations to improve the performance of fidelity-constrained entanglement routing.

Proposed Solution and Contribution

We propose and investigate, for the first time to the best of our knowledge, the problem of link configuration for fidelity-constrained routing and purification (LC-FCRP) in quantum networks, which aims to guarantee the fidelity of distributed entanglements by jointly tuning link configuration and entanglement routing with purification [13]. We formulate a simplified version of the FCRP problem as a Mixed Integer Linear Programming (MILP) model, assuming that link fidelities can be configured within a finite set, jointly optimizing the link configuration and purification decisions. We design a novel link configuration algorithm based on a shortest-path-based fidelity determination (SPFD) algorithm w/o Bayesian Optimization, which can be applied on top of existing ER algorithms.

5 Conclusion

In summary, we investigated resource allocation algorithms for green, resilient, and secure future optical networks. We began by discussing the state-of-the-art studies on energy efficiency, resiliency, and security for future optical networks and analyzed the corresponding key challenges. To address these challenges, we studied novel resource allocation algorithms for future optical networks. In particular, we focused on enhancing energy efficiency with novel optical-transmission approaches, improving network resiliency with proactive and reactive strategies, and enhancing network security with quantum technologies. The comprehensive results demonstrate the effectiveness of the proposed solutions to improve the energy efficiency, resiliency, and security for future optical networks.

Competing Interests The authors have no conflicts of interest to declare that are relevant to the content of this chapter.

Ethics Approval No ethical approval was required for this study.

Acknowledgements This work was supported by the Italian Ministry of University and Research (MUR) and the European Union (EU) under the PON/REACT project.

References

1. L. Al-Tarawneh, A. Alqatawneh, A. Tahat, O. Saraereh, Evolution of optical networks: from legacy networks to next-generation networks. IEEE/Opt. J. Opt. Commun. **44**(s1), s955–s970 (2024)
2. L. Chen et al., *Report on Post-quantum Cryptography* (US Department of Commerce, National Institute of Standards and Technology, 2016)
3. T. Zami, B. Lavigne, Optimal deployments of 400 gb/s multihaul cfp2-dco transponders in transparent ipowdm core networks, in *Optical Fiber Communication Conference* (2022)
4. Q. Zhang, A. Morea, P. Layec, M. Ibrahimi, F. Musumeci, M. Tornatore, Power-consumption analysis for different ipowdm network architectures with zr/zr+ and long-haul muxponders. IEEE/Optica J. Opt. Commun. Netw. **16**(12), 1189–1203 (2024)
5. Q. Zhang, P. Layec, A. May, A. Morea, A. Attarpour, M. Tornatore, Cost and power-consumption analysis for power profile monitoring with multiple monitors per link in optical networks, *Optical Switching and Networking*, p. 100813 (2025)
6. G. Le, S. Ferdousi, A. Marotta, S. Xu, Y. Hirota, Y. Awaji, M. Tornatore, B. Mukherjee, Survivable virtual network mapping with content connectivity against multiple link failures in optical metro networks. IEEE/Opt. J. Opt. Commun. Netw. **12**(11), 301–311 (2020)
7. Q. Zhang, O. Ayoub, R. Wang, E. Viadana, F. Musumeci, M. Tornatore, Capacity sharing for survivable virtual network mapping against double-link failures. *IEEE Trans. Netw. Serv. Manage.* **22**(4), 3003–3015 (2025)
8. R. Wang, Q. Zhang, J. Zhang, Z. Gu, M. Ibrahimi, H. Yu, B. Zhang, F. Musumeci, Y. Ji, M. Tornatore, Multi-failure localization in high-degree roadm-based optical networks using rules-informed neural networks. IEEE J. Sel. Areas Commun. **43**(5), 1738–1754 (2025)
9. Q. Zhang, O. Ayoub, J. Wu, F. Musumeci, G. Li, M. Tornatore, Progressive slice recovery with guaranteed slice connectivity after massive failures. IEEE/ACM Trans. Netw. **30**(2), 826–839 (2021)
10. Y. Cao, Y. Zhao, Q. Wang, J. Zhang, S.X. Ng, L. Hanzo, The evolution of quantum key distribution networks: on the road to the qinternet. IEEE Commun. Surv. Tutor. **24**(2), 839–894 (2022)
11. Q. Zhang, O. Ayoub, A. Gatto, J. Wu, F. Musumeci, M. Tornatore, Routing, channel, key-rate, and time-slot assignment for qkd in optical networks. IEEE Trans. Netw. Serv. Manag. **21**(1), 148–160 (2024)
12. G. Vardoyan, S. Wehner, Quantum network utility maximization, in *IEEE International Conference on Quantum Computing and Engineering (QCE)*, vol. 1 (IEEE, 2023), pp. 1238–1248
13. Q. Zhang, N. Di Cicco, M. Ibrahimi, R.C. Almeida, A. Gatto, R. Boutaba, M. Tornatore, Link configuration for fidelity-constrained entanglement routing in quantum networks, in *IEEE Conference on Computer Communications (INFOCOM)* (IEEE, 2025)

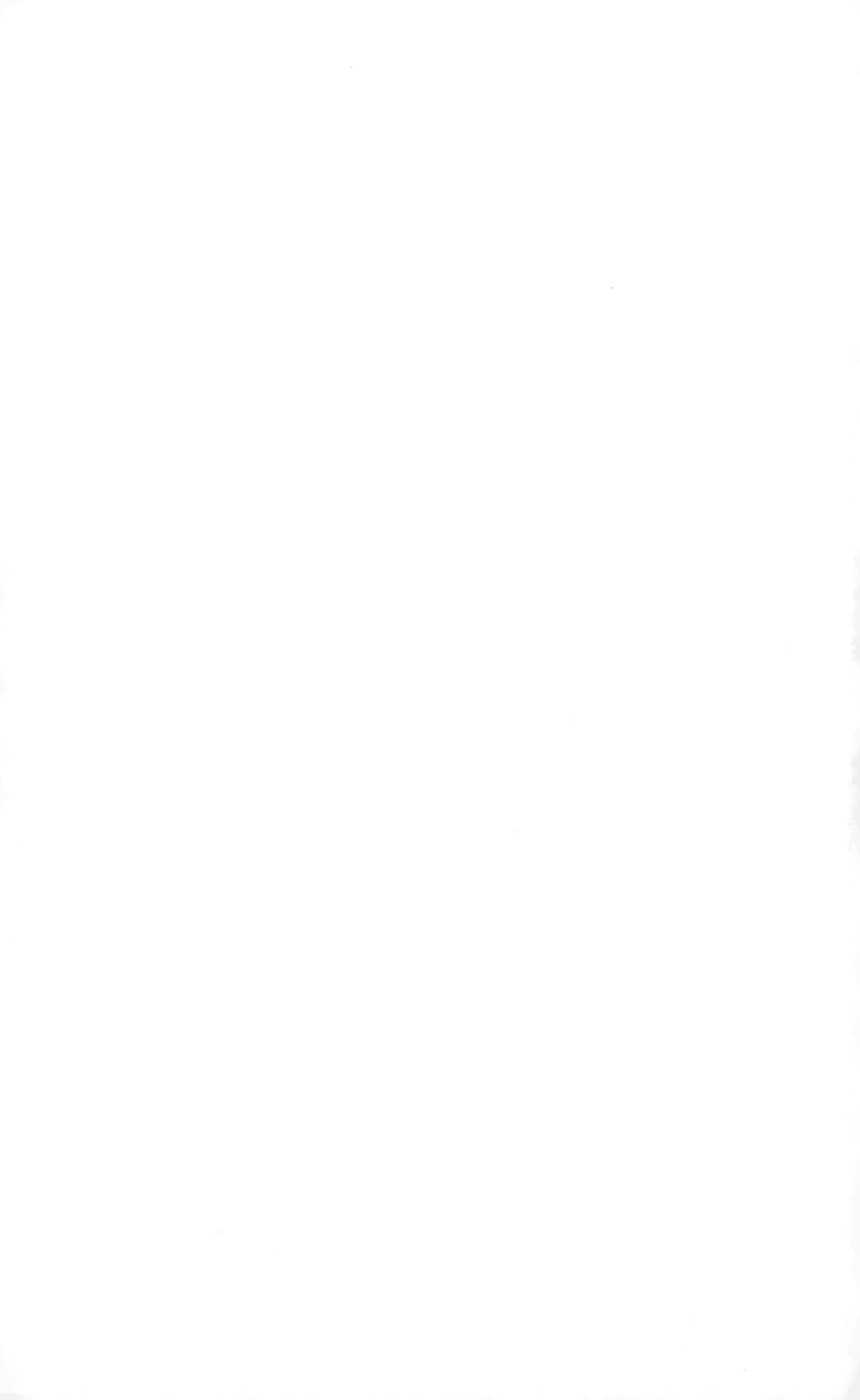

GPSR Compliance
The European Union's (EU) General Product Safety Regulation (GPSR) is a set
of rules that requires consumer products to be safe and our obligations to
ensure this.

If you have any concerns about our products, you can contact us on

ProductSafety@springernature.com

In case Publisher is established outside the EU, the EU authorized
representative is:

Springer Nature Customer Service Center GmbH
Europaplatz 3
69115 Heidelberg, Germany